Keto for Women Over 50

2 Books in 1:

Your Essential Guide to Ketogenic Diet and Meal Prep for Beginners. Easy and Quick Recipes to Reset Your Metabolism, Boost Your Energy, and Heal Your Body. Bonus: 30-Day Meal Plan

© **Copyright 2019 - All rights reserved.**

The content contained within this book may not be reproduced, duplicated or transmitted without direct written permission from the author or the publisher.

Under no circumstances will any blame or legal responsibility be held against the publisher, or author, for any damages, reparation, or monetary loss due to the information contained within this book. Either directly or indirectly.

Legal Notice:

This book is copyright protected. This book is only for personal use. You cannot amend, distribute, sell, use, quote or paraphrase any part, or the content within this book, without the consent of the author or publisher.

Disclaimer Notice:

Please note the information contained within this document is for educational and entertainment purposes only. All effort has been executed to present accurate, up to date, and reliable, complete information. No warranties of any kind are declared or implied. Readers acknowledge that the author is not engaging in the rendering of legal, financial, medical or professional advice. The content within this book has been derived from various sources. Please consult a licensed professional before attempting any techniques outlined in this book.

By reading this document, the reader agrees that under no circumstances is the author responsible for any losses, direct or indirect, which are incurred as a result of the use of the information contained within this document, including, but not limited to, — errors, omissions, or inaccuracies.

Table of Contents

Keto Diet for Women Over 50

Introduction 13

Chapter 1: The Keto Diet for Beginners 17

Chapter 2: Starting the Ketogenic Diet 25

Chapter 3: Keto Diet Nutrition: 34

30 Day Meal Plan 34

    Day 1: Scrambled Eggs 35

    Day 2: Pesto Chicken Casserole 36

    Day 3: Keto Meat Pie 38

    Day 4: Keto Carbonara 41

    Day 5: Keto Bread 44

    Day 6: Keto Pizza 46

    Day 7: Keto Frittata 48

    Day 8: Keto BLT 50

    Day 9: Keto Coconut Porridge 53

    Day 10: Keto Tex-Mex Casserole 55

    Day 11: Chorizo with Creamed Green Cabbage 57

    Day 12: Keto Mushroom Omelet 59

Day 13: Keto Lasagna 61

Day 14: Turkey with Cream Cheese Sauce 65

Day 15: Boiled Eggs With Mayo 67

Day 16: Keto Beef Stew 69

Day 17: Keto Stuffed Cabbage 71

Day 18: Keto Mac and Cheese 74

Day 19: Keto Fried Chicken 77

Day 20: Keto Broccoli Salad 79

Day 21: Keto Meatballs 81

Day 22: Keto Garlic Rosemary Pork Chops 83

Day 23: Keto Cheesy Bacon Ranch Chicken 85

Day 24: Keto Bacon Sushi 87

Day 26: Keto Chicken Parmesan 91

Day 27: Keto Meatloaf 94

Day 28: Keto Garlicky Lemon Mahi-Mahi 96

Day 29: Keto Philly Cheesesteak Lettuce Wraps 98

Day 30: Keto Tuscan Butter Shrimp 100

Chapter 4: Hormone and Diabetes Support on Keto ... 102

Chapter 5: Keto Tips and Tricks 110

Chapter 6: How to Reset your Metabolism 120

Chapter 7: Keto FAQs 128

Chapter 8: Doing Keto as a Woman Over 50 135

Chapter 9: How to Have More Energy **142**

Chapter 10: Best Exercises to Lose Weight **149**

Forearm Plan *152*

Modified Push-Up *153*

Basic Squat *153*

Stability Ball Chest Fly *153*

Stability Ball Tricep Kick Back *154*

Shoulder Overhead Press *155*

Stability Ball Overhead Pull *155*

Stability Ball Side Leg Lift *156*

Single-Leg Hamstring Bridge *156*

Bird Dog *156*

Conclusion **157**

Meal Prep for Beginners

Introduction 163
Chapter 1: What is Prepping? 165
Chapter 2: 10 Reasons Why You Should Meal Prep 168
   Better Control on Portions 169
   Save Money 169
   Improve Your Skills in Cooking 170
   Eliminate Hidden Calories 171
   Save Time 171
   Better Results from Workouts 172
   Come Home to a Nice Meal 172
   Variety In Your Meals 173
   Increase Your Willpower 173
   No More Food Wastage 174
Chapter 3: Tips and Tricks to Make Meal Prepping Easier 175
   Don't Stuff Too Many Things At a Time 176
   Be Organized 176
   Keep Each Food Group in Mind 177
   Get Quality Meal Prep Containers 178
   Your Pantry Should Be Well Stocked 179
   Always Keep Enough Spices and Herbs on Hand 180
   Make Time for Meal Planning 181
   Always Take a Shopping List to the Grocery Store 181
   Repurpose Leftovers 183
   Enjoy the Process 183
Chapter 4: Easy Meal Prep Recipes 185
   Breakfast 186

Freezer Breakfast Sandwiches 186
Oatmeal Breakfast Bites.. 189
Turmeric Scrambled Eggs 191
Frozen Yogurt Granola Cups 193
Sweet Potato Breakfast Bowl 195
Choco Chip Oatmeal Squares 197
Bacon Quiche With Potato Crust.. 199
Scrambled Tofu Breakfast Burritos...202
Avocado Quinoa Frittatas 206

Lunch..209
Sweet and Spicy Tempeh Bowls 209
Vegetable Barley Soup... 213
Roasted Vegetables and Sausage.. 216
Jerk Chicken With Black Beans and Pineapple Salsa 220
Black-Eyed Peas Meal Prep 223
Black-Eyed Peas...226

Dinner 229
Honey Glazed Meatballs 229
Soy Glazed Chicken With Garlic Noodles 232
Soy Glazed Chicken 234
Beef and Broccoli... 237
BBQ Baked Zucchini and Salmon 241
Thai Coconut Quinoa Bowls 244

Salads and Vegetables 249
Artichoke and Avocado Pasta Salad.......................................249
Apple Arugula and Turkey Salad in a Jar 251
Summertime Slaw 254
Zucchini and Tomato Spaghetti 256
White Bean Salad...259
Lentil Bolognese 262

    Kale, Lemon, and White Bean Soup 265

    Broccoli Quinoa Casserole 268

Fish and Seafood *270*

    Shrimp Fajita 270

    Salmon Cobb Salad 273

    Asparagus Shrimp Stir Fry 275

    Shrimp Boil Skillet 278

    Tuna Salad 281

    Shrimp Stir Fry 283

Healthy Snacks and Desserts *285*

    Frozen Banana Bites 285

    Italian Kale Chips 287

    Apple and Quinoa Bars 289

    Avocado Toast 291

    Tuna Protein Box 293

    Puffed Quinoa Bars 295

    Roasted Broccoli 297

    Tuna Patties 299

    Rosemary Keto Crackers 301

Chapter 5: 30-Day Meal Prep Plan for 303
Weight Loss 303

Week 1 .... *304*

    Breakfast – Low Carb Waffles 304

    Lunch – Avocado Basil Shrimp Wraps 306

    Snacks – Peanut Butter Granola Bars 309

    Dinner – Beef and Broccoli 311

Week 2 ....*312*

    Breakfast – Avocado Quinoa Frittatas 312

    Lunch – Collard Wrap Bento Boxes 313

    Snacks – Chocolate Barks 315

    Dinner – Zoodle Ramen 317

  Week 3 .... *320*

    Breakfast – Egg Muffins 320

    Lunch – Steak Salad 322

    Snacks – Mango Sorbet 324

    Dinner – Lentil Bolognese 326

  Week 4 .... *327*

    Breakfast – Strawberry Overnight Oats 327

    Lunch – One Pan Salmon and Asparagus 329

    Snacks – Pumpkin Pie Balls 331

    Dinner – California Roll Sushi Bowls 333

Chapter 6: Healthy Meals to Prep and Go 336

  Sheet Pan Cashew Chicken 336

  Almond Flour Pancakes 340

  Asian Lemon Chicken 342

  Berry Fruit Salad 345

  Deli Style Protein Box 347

  Simple Breakfast Meal Prep 350

  Mason Jar Chicken Salad 353

  Taco Meal Prep Bowl 356

  Greek Chicken Meal Prep Bowls 358

Chapter 7: Grocery Shopping Tips for Meal Preppers . 362

  Stick to One Supermarket *362*

  Make a Store Map of Your Own *363*

  Have a Digital Meal List *363*

  Be Aware of the Sales *364*

Conclusion 365

Keto Diet for Women Over 50

An Essential Guide to Ketogenic Diet and Weight Loss!

Easy Keto Recipes to Reset Your Metabolism, Boost your Energy, and Heal Your Body

Bonus: 30-Day Meal Plan

Jason Watchers

Introduction

Congratulations on purchasing *Keto Diet for Women over 50,* and thank you for doing so.

Whether you don't know the first thing about Keto or you want to clear up some of the things you've heard about it, *Keto Diet for Women over 50* has the answers you are looking for.

If you have been searching for an all-in-one guide to show you how to do Keto the right way, you need not look any further. *Keto Diet for Women* over 50 covers it all: I'll show you how to reset your metabolism while eating foods you already love. Women all over the world are waking up to the power of Keto and using it to reach their goal weight, revive their energy levels, and get back their glowing, youthful skin.

And Keto doesn't end there—while most women start Keto to lose weight, I'll uncover the hidden truth about Keto and how it heals your body at the cellular level. Not only will you get more practical knowledge from this book than any other, but all of it is backed by scientific data—all in one place.

In the first chapter, we will go through all the basics of Keto. There is a lot of buzz about Keto these days, but unfortunately, there is a lot of wrong information about it too. We will answer all the "he said, she said" about Keto in this book by getting the facts straight and diving deep into well-researched facts and studies of what Keto actually does to our body and our overall health.

All of the information contained in these pages has been heavily fact-checked to ensure you are getting only the most accurate information. That way, you can endeavor on your personal journey to change your body, regain the energy of your youth, and never worry about your body image again.

This book prioritizes the most important and practical information about Keto. I put it at the top of every chapter and section; you don't have to dig deep in the chapters to get the most important information. However, the smaller details are still included so you can learn as much about Keto as possible.

We go through the perfect mix of Keto basics and finer details of Keto. The more invested you get in this diet and lifestyle, the more you will want to dive into these finer details. But in the beginning, you may want to read just for the fundamentals. You can always expand your Keto knowledge later.

At the end of the day, this is not a science book: it is a book with the explicit and only aim of helping you apply the science of Keto to your real life. As such, I give you all the up-to-date and well-researched facts, but in an easily digestible manner.

If you haven't heard anything about Keto before, the first thing you need to know is its goal. Many people around the world—from women to men, from old to young—use Keto to help their bodies lose weight, to trigger the process of autophagy and the health benefits that come with it, and to give their skin a youthful glow.

But no matter what your goals are, from a scientific standpoint, there is only one goal: to trigger something called Ketosis in your system.

I give you all the most important biological facts so you can see for yourself that Keto is not just a trend—it is deeply rooted in science. But most of the book is not about science. It is about how to get started with Keto, particularly if you are a woman over 50.

You won't find a better book on Keto for someone like you. This is the only one that will help you do Keto the right way, so you see the results from it as soon as possible.

As you flip through these pages, you will see that I spend a lot of time going through the mistakes that Keto beginners make with the Keto lifestyle. The book focuses on these common mistakes because you can learn from them and avoid making them yourself.

You will find no better source for the science of Keto, how to incorporate Keto into your daily life, and the nitty-gritty details of the diet itself. We get into the weeds with how Keto affects hormones, how it affects women over 50 in particular, and how Keto can reset your metabolism.

There are plenty of books on this subject on the market, thanks again for choosing this one! Every effort was made to ensure it is full of as much useful information as possible. Please enjoy!

Chapter 1:
The Keto Diet for Beginners

If you made it this far into your research on Keto, you've already heard a lot of things about it. Many of them will turn out to be untrue because, unfortunately, there is a lot of misinformation floating around on the topic.

This chapter addresses all of these misconceptions and arms you with up-to-date, accurate facts on Keto so you can start the diet with confidence. Let's begin with the basic science that makes Keto work.

The ultimate goal of following the Ketogenic diet is to activate a process called Ketosis.

You probably already know the basic idea of Keto, but we'll still go over it for purposes of clarification. The Keto diet is a pattern of eating that causes your body to burn fat as a source of energy. It does this by triggering the process of Ketosis.

During Ketosis, your body releases chemicals in your body called Ketones. Ketones come from your liver, but your liver only produces them if you are not consuming many carbs. When you consume a lot of carbs, your body has no reason to go through Ketosis, since your body is spending so much time digesting the carbs instead.

This is why people who do Keto don't only lose weight—they report a distinct increase in their energy, too. With Ketones flowing through their veins, and with their bodies using fat as an additional source of energy, they feel refreshed.

This brings us to the topic of autophagy, a microbiological that goes hand-in-hand with Keto. Not only will Keto get you to lose weight and feel more energetic, but you will feel unmistakably refreshed, and it is all thanks to autophagy.

Autophagy is what your cells do to clean out waste. Your cells produce all kinds of microscopic waste. This includes proteins they are no longer using, organelles that are too damaged, and materials that came from outside the cell.

Your cells trigger autophagy when they have no food source other than cellular waste. That's why the most direct method of getting your cells to enter advanced autophagy is through fasting—that is, not eating for some period of time.

Another method of triggering autophagy is by following the Keto diet.

Keto deprives your body of carbs. It is important that you have significantly less carbs in your body to trigger Ketosis, but there's another reason, too. Carbs are the nutrient that your body spends the most time breaking down. Because of this, following Keto is a great way to trigger autophagy. You can get the positive effects of both Ketosis and autophagy by simply limiting your carb intake.

My advice is to follow an eating schedule where you don't eat for at least seven hours during the day. That way, your fasting will trigger advanced autophagy while you also trigger Ketosis with your diet. In addition, the low carb intake from Keto will increase your autophagy body even further.

Understanding why people rely on Keto to lose weight and trigger autophagy is easier when you look at a lifestyle that is the opposite of Keto. Many Americans have carbs as the source of 50% of their calories. When you eat a lot of carbs, you create a backup in your digestive system.

It takes approximately four hours for your system to digest a low-carb meal. Your cells won't start autophagy until they have no outside food to get energy from. That means as long as your body is digesting these carbs, you will not go through autophagy.

We always act like your fast starts the moment you stop eating, but from the perspective of your cells, the fast doesn't really start until four hours after you stop eating. That means a 7-hour fast in the middle of the day only really means a 3-hour fast for your cells, during which time they will rely on autophagy to get energy.

Now, let's bring carbs into the picture. It changes things drastically: when you eat a meal high in carbs, it doesn't take 4 hours for your body to break it down: it takes 8.

You might eat a high-carb meal and think you are fasting for 7 hours after that, but you are not actually getting a fast in at all. The entire time between your meals, your body is still digesting the carbs you ate. You may as well not have done the 7-hour fast at all.

This is where Keto and autophagy work together. You can rely on healthy fats for energy that our bodies burn through Ketosis instead of carbs. Meanwhile, your low carb intake makes your body go into autophagy much faster after you stop eating. Keto lends itself very well to autophagy.

Women around the world are learning about autophagy. That's because triggering autophagy helps them achieve many of the goals women use Keto for: to reach their goal weight, to boost their energy, and to have healthier skin, just to name a few.

Women trigger autophagy through a variety of methods, and Keto is only one of them. The most popular method is intermittent fasting. Intermittent fasting is mostly the same as your traditional fast, but instead of not eating for a day or more at a time, you simply fast for a set number of hours every day. Earlier I recommended the 7-hour fast, and this would fall under the umbrella of an intermittent fast.

The other method is exercise. Strength training triggers autophagy as directly as fasting does. Our muscles go through tears that are impossible to see with the human eye; the only way for our body to repair these tears is through autophagy. When we exercise a few times a week, we enable the cells in our bodies to go through autophagy as much as possible.

The Keto diet is another way to stimulate autophagy. However, there is one common misunderstanding about autophagy: some women think autophagy is either "on" or "off." The fact is, our bodies are always going through autophagy somewhere. So when we say to trigger autophagy, we really mean to reach advanced autophagy. Maintenance-mode autophagy is the kind that is always going on somewhere in your body, while advanced autophagy only happens when you fast, exercise, or follow the Keto diet. From this point on, read "autophagy" as meaning "advanced autophagy."

We can trigger advanced autophagy through any of the three methods listed so far, but I recommend the Keto diet as your primary method. Ideally, you still use fasting and exercise to make your autophagy even more potent; the last chapter tells you which exercises women over 50 can do to help them maximize autophagy. But the Keto diet will do the most to optimize the autophagy that your system will already go through.

There is one key reason for this, and it is about practicality. Women tend to find it easier to change their diet than to avoid eating during big chunks of the day. Intermittent fasting helps women trigger autophagy too, but intermittent fasting is harder to keep up than a change of diet.

This is why I recommend Keto over intermittent fasting. But if you are able to combine the two of them, you will see even faster results.

Autophagy detoxifies your cells of waste; Ketosis introduces Ketones in your system that burn fat for energy—leading to the Ketones appearing in your system.

Women have a similar misconception about Ketosis that they have with autophagy. With autophagy, they think they are turning it "on" with fasting, and it is "off" when they are not fasting. In reality, they are triggering advanced autophagy with fasting, but some autophagy was always there.

The same idea goes for Ketosis. Without Ketosis, your body will still burn fat for energy. That's why people are still able to lose weight through exercise and caloric restriction alone: you can still burn fat without the Keto diet; it is just a lot slower. Keto is how you can burn fat for energy at a much faster rate.

But now that you know you can speed up the process by eating Ketogenic foods, it doesn't make sense not to follow it anymore. It is hard to go back to your old eating habits when you know you can lose weight fast with Keto and autophagy.

We all know that the real reason Keto is popular is not for health reasons. It is because Keto is a way of losing weight that actually works. Not only does it work, but women say it works much more quickly than any other method of dieting they have tried.

Fasting helps women lose weight too, but the fact is, most people are not able to stick with a routine of not eating for seven hours or more every day. Fasting gets you a similar level of health benefits as Keto, but it is harder to keep up with.

Anyone can do Keto; what holds women back isn't that it is particularly hard to do for a few days. Sticking with fasting in the long-term is what makes it hard as a practical way of losing weight. The lack of practicality of fasting is why it is quickly losing favor as a weight-loss strategy, while more and more women are turning to Keto.

You will learn everything you need to know to be a Keto pro as you read through these chapters. Now that you know the basics by the back of your hand, you are almost ready to move on to the next chapter. Chapter 2 focuses on how you actually get started with Keto once you understand what you are getting into.

Before you get there, I have a word of caution. Some women will follow the Keto diet to a tee but miss this one crucial thing.

Missing this one thing will throw off the purpose of the diet entirely, and it will even prevent them from getting the benefits they were looking for in Keto. That means it is very important for you to understand where these women go wrong.

I am referring to the principle of "calories in, calories out" that applies to every diet—not just Keto. You may replace all your calories from carbs with calories from healthy fats just as you are supposed to, but you still won't lose weight if you are eating too many calories in total.

It only makes sense: if you are consuming too many calories without burning them off with exercise, even with very few of them coming from carbs, you will still find yourself not losing weight. Please keep this in mind as you start up your Keto journey.

Chapter 2:
Starting the Ketogenic Diet

You have already done much of the work to change over to a healthy lifestyle now that you know how Keto works. Of course, to make the most of the knowledge, you still have a lot to learn.

While the last chapter gave you the theoretical side of Keto, this one tells you how to take action on the information you have. You'll also learn some of the common mistakes new Keto followers make and how to avoid them.

You'll learn how to be proactive in your approach by keeping a log of your daily eating habits. Your Keto journal will make sure you are making real progress.

Before we cover the common mistakes, women make with Keto. First, we need to look a little deeper into Ketosis itself. As you know, practitioners of this diet are doing it as a way to trigger Ketosis.

Ketosis is the biological process in which your liver produces Ketones that cause your body to burn fat for energy. You get this to happen by depriving your body of its usual source of energy: carbs.

But it is actually a little more complicated than that, despite what other Keto books might have you believe. This is a way of explaining Ketosis that understandably simplifies it, but by doing so, it ignores some of the important components of Ketosis.

First of all, it isn't quite true that your body burns carbs for energy. Instead, your body uses those carbs to burn something else for energy: glucose. Glucose is the sugar that comes from the food that you eat.

It is different from the sugar you have in your pantry. Your digestive system breaks down everything you eat into its most basic parts so it can use the food for energy. Glucose is what comes out of this process of digestion. You could say it is the basic source of energy for your body.

When you put your body through Ketosis, this is a way of getting your system to use Ketones for the job that carbs would normally do. Meanwhile, the Ketones themselves get your body to burn more fat.

What makes Keto attractive to many women is the fact that it uses biological mechanisms already present in your body to burn fat. You aren't taking a pill to lose weight that won't actually work. Your body can already go through Ketosis without any medication; all you have to do is follow the Keto diet.

It isn't exactly true when people say you put your body through Ketosis to get these Ketones to burn fat. The job of

Ketones is not to burn fat, but to aid in the process of burning through glucose.

When you don't eat a lot of carbs, carbs don't do the job of burning your glucose anymore. Instead, your liver produces Ketones that burn fat.

There is a lot of misinformation that spreads because people learn about Keto from word-of-mouth or other unreliable sources instead of learning about it directly from a book.

Many people get the false impression that the only thing we do in Keto is lower our carb intake. They do not think there is any more to it than that. Of course, it is a major part of Keto. But if it is the only part of the Keto diet you are following, you are not going about it in a healthy way.

That's because the other vitally important aspect of the Ketogenic diet is eating healthy fats. Make sure you get that into your mind because it is extremely important.

If you aren't getting a lot of healthy fats into your diet, and you aren't eating many carbs, you are not doing Keto. This is simply bad for your body. When you eat few carbs, you are already depriving your body of something it normally has, putting your cells in a state of stress that will trigger autophagy while simultaneously—and most importantly—triggering Ketosis.

The Ketosis will indeed cause an influx of Ketones that burn through your fat. However, if you don't have healthy fats to burn for energy, you will end up hurting yourself.

Everyone needs energy in order to live. Someone who deprives themselves of carbs and fats will only end up hurting themselves. When you dramatically decrease your carb intake in Keto, make sure you replace those calories with healthy, nutrient-rich foods like vegetables and sources of healthy fats.

By this point, you will experience the subjective changes that come with changing to a Keto lifestyle. You will feel a surge of energy, notice significant weight loss, and even feel cleansed through the natural process of autophagy. You will notice all of these things as long as you closely follow the directions provided here.

However, you may be looking for a more tangible way of seeing your progress in Keto. There is a way you can figure out how strong your Ketosis is, and all it requires is a blood sugar tester.

This may not be for everyone. For some people, the subjective difference they feel in their energy and the weight loss itself will be enough for them to know they are in Ketosis. They might not like the idea of having to draw blood to test their Ketosis with the blood sugar tester. Maybe the price of the blood sugar tester isn't worth it; it isn't exactly expensive, but it isn't exactly cheap, either. This is completely fine; if you feel like you are getting what you need from Keto, that should be enough for you.

Others want to know for a fact that Ketosis is the reason for their weight loss. They want to be certain that their other lifestyle changes are not the reason for their weight loss.

There is a method for you to be more certain if you are going through significant Ketosis. You just need a blood sugar tester to calculate your glucose-Ketone index.

The Ketone-glucose index will tell you whether you are going through significant Ketosis. It will also indicate whether you are going through advanced autophagy.

First, purchase the blood sugar. After that, you want to wait until you have been following Keto for a long enough time. I recommend waiting until you have been on Keto for two weeks. If you have only been doing Keto for a week, this test will not be accurate.

In fact, you will want to be sure you have been consistently doing Keto for two weeks—without cheating the requirements—before taking this blood sugar test. Only then should you take the results seriously.

After you are on Keto for two weeks, you will plug the numbers from the test into a specific formula. This formula will give you your glucose-Ketone index. The meter will give you a numeral for glucose and another for Ketone.

For blood sugar meters that use mmol/L, as most do, you will have to divide the glucose numeral by 18. You will not have to divide by 18 if the blood sugar test uses mg/dL, because this part of the equation is only to get us to use the correct units.

Once the conversion is done, the next thing you do is divide your glucose value by the Ketone value. You can remember which is which from the name of the index: glucose-Ketone. Start with your glucose, and divide it by your Ketone. After that, you will have your glucose-Ketone index. It is as simple as that. From there, it is only a matter of interpreting this number and knowing what it means.

As a general rule, you would like a glucose-Ketone index from 6 to 9. This indicates that your body is going through significant Ketosis. Now let's talk about where you definitely don't want to fall on the glucose-Ketone index. If your index is lower than 3, this is where you may be going through some stage of cancer and may even experience seizures.

Of course, you won't be in this range of the index unless you already know you have cancer or some other serious condition, so this isn't something you need to think much about.

On the less extreme end of things, if your glucose-Ketone index goes from 3 to 6, that is an indicator that you suffer from obesity. It is unlikely that you will have an index in this range if you are only overweight, especially on the lower end.

If you are overweight and not obese and you find yourself on the lower end of this 3 to 6 range, you may be in danger of slipping from overweight territory into obesity, so keep that in mind.

This is certainly not where you want to land when you put yourself through Ketosis, but that doesn't mean you aren't going through Ketosis in this range. The glucose-Ketone index may be the most objective metric we have, but there are a lot of different factors that can come into play.

If you are already overweight and follow the Keto diet consistently and correctly for two weeks, you may still be somewhere in the 3 to 6 range. You may just have to wait until you lose some more weight before you see your index increase and go above 6.

An index above 9 is not desirable; it simply means you are not going through significant Ketosis. You will have to stick with it for longer to see this number drop.

Ultimately, you want your index to fall somewhere between 6 and 9. For a woman seeking to trigger Ketosis, this is the ideal index to have. Since this index tells you that you are going through significant Ketosis, it comes with a lot of good news. When you fall within this range, you will find it relatively easy to maintain the weight you have or lose weight if you aren't content with where you are.

As I said, you need to look at this index with some skepticism. Just because it is the most tangible way to look at the progression of your Ketosis, that doesn't make it perfect. Even if your index is between 6 and 9, that doesn't mean you should blindly accept that to mean you are going through Ketosis. Unfortunately, it just isn't that easy.

You should look for subjective signs as well as your index to determine if your Ketosis is significant. These signs include the health of your skin, whether you are losing weight, and how much energy you feel you have every day.

In the same way, an index outside of 6 and 9 doesn't mean you definitely are not going through Ketosis. With the many factors that go into it, it could just be the last thing you ate.

The reason for the variability is because blood sugar fluctuates a lot. Your blood sugar level at one moment won't be the same as the blood sugar level you have at the next.

When you use the index, use it together with some plain common sense. Ask yourself if you feel better, whether your skin looks better, and look at the number on the scale. These will all be as useful as the index.

Don't look at the glucose-Ketone index as the only way of measuring how healthy you are. You could fall between 6 and 9 and not be healthy. If you fall outside 6 and 9 from time to time, you might still be healthy, too. You should take all of these things into consideration.

Finally, I suggest you keep a journal with all of this information in it. Mark down the days you go to the gym, what exercises you do, and how much time you spend there. Mark down what Keto-friendly foods you are eating, and write down their carb, fat, protein, and calorie content.

The next chapter goes through thirty recipes you can follow, so you have a month's worth of foods that all fit into the Keto diet. I am positive you will love eating these delicious meals.

Chapter 3:
Keto Diet Nutrition:
30 Day Meal Plan

Followers of Keto don't have to stop eating the foods they love. We cover 30 days of delicious meals that all abide by the rules of the Ketogenic diet. These include scrambled eggs, pesto chicken casserole, meat pie, Keto carbonara, and much, much more.

These recipes were selected for two main reasons: because they follow the requirements of Keto while also being simple to prepare and cook.

Day 1: Scrambled Eggs

With Keto-friendly scrambled eggs, you just add butter to eggs. It can't get simpler than that. This makes the best breakfast you could ask for while staying within the confines of Keto. There's no more pleasant way to wake up your taste buds than a plate of scrumptious scrambled eggs. Keto scrambled eggs pair well with a hot cup of coffee, but skip on the milk in that coffee, as milk has high carb content.

Ingredients:

- 1 oz. butter
- 2 eggs
- Spices as desired

Directions:

1. Put eggs in the bowl, whisking them, and adding your desired spices.
2. Wait for the butter to melt down on the pan. Be sure not to burn your butter; you want it to melt without getting burnt.
3. Place eggs in the skillet and stir occasionally until they are cooked your preferred way. Depending on how you like to cook your eggs, it is entirely up to you how long this is.

Day 2: Pesto Chicken Casserole

This one is a Mediterranean classic that is easy to make. Keto practitioners want to eat pesto that is low in carbs. Other than that, there's no difference between Keto pesto chicken casserole and normal pesto chicken casserole.

Ingredients:

- 1 pound of chicken
- 5 tablespoons pesto
- 5 ounces diced feta cheese
- 1 finely chopped clove of garlic
- Spices as desired
- 3 ounces pitted olives
- 2 tablespoons margarine
- 1 and 1/4 cups whipped cream

Directions:

1. Set your oven to 400°F.
2. Slice your chicken into small chunks. Add desired spices. If you're unsure what to add, you can just use classics like salt or pepper.

3. Put oil and butter in your skillet. Cook the small bits of chicken on a heat setting between high and medium until they turn golden brown.

4. You can either use pesto you bought at the store, or you can make your own. Combine it with the whipped cream in your bowl.

5. Put the small bits of chicken together with the olives, garlic, and cheese. After that, mix in the pesto and whipped cream mix you made a moment ago.

6. Cook in the oven for twenty to thirty minutes. When it is done, it will turn bubbly. The edges of the dish should be a light brown, not golden brown.

Day 3: Keto Meat Pie

Everyone likes meat pie. Some say it is too traditional and not innovative enough, but it is good to stick with what you know from time to time. Traditional meals are especially useful for helping us approach a new diet.

Ingredients:

- Pie crust
- 3/4 cup flour
- 4 tablespoons coconut flour
- 1 teaspoons baking powder
- 1 egg
- A dash of salt
- 4 tablespoons of water
- 3 tablespoons of melted olive oil

Topping:

- 8 ounces of cottage cheese
- 7 ounces of shredded cheese

Filling:

- Half a yellow onion, chopped into thin pieces
- 1 garlic clove, chopped into thin pieces
- 2 tablespoons of butter or olive oil
- 1 and 3/4 pounds of ground beef
- 1 tablespoons of dried oregano
- Desired spices
- 4 tablespoons of tomato paste
- Half a cup of water

Directions:

1. Set the oven to 350°F

2. Cook onion and garlic in the butter over moderate heat for 2-3 minutes, and stop when the onion softens up. Put in the beef and continue cooking. Put in the oregano. Add your desired spices.

3. Mix in tomato paste, then water. Reduce the heat and allow for simmering up to half an hour. As it simmers, you can focus on putting together the dough for the

crust.

4. Put together the crust ingredients in a food processor. Process the food as long as it takes until the dough turns into a ball. You don't necessarily need a food processor, though; you can get the same thing done with a fork. Just be sure to be thorough.

5. Put the parchment paper in a well-greased springform pan; this will help make it easier to take out the pie when it is finished. Spread the dough all the way to the very edges of the pan. You may utilize a spatula or your fingers as long as they are lubricated in oil enough. Once the crust is shaped to the pan, poke with a fork.

6. Pre-bake the crust for ten to fifteen minutes. Take it out of the oven and put the meat in the crust. Mix the cottage cheese and shredded cheese all together. Place it on top of the pie.

7. Cook on the lower rack for half an hour; by this time, the dish should be a golden brown color.

Day 4: Keto Carbonara

You can start using zucchini pasta for all your pasta needs without having to worry about the carb content of traditional pasta ever again. The crunch of the bacon combined with the smoothness of this Italian cuisine will convince you to make this dish again and again.

Ingredients:

- 1 and 1/4 cups whipped cream
- 1 tablespoons of butter
- 10 ounces of bacon
- 1/4 cups of mayo
- Desired spices
- 2 pounds of zucchini
- 4 egg yolks
- 3 ounces of parmesan

Directions:

1. Pour the whipped cream into a pan. Boil it over a moderately high heat setting. Turn the heat down to medium-low, letting it boil for some minutes.

2. Use a big pan to melt the butter over moderate heat. Put the bacon into the pan, cooking it until it is crisp. Put your bacon aside. Don't move the fat outside the pan, but instead keep it warm, not turning up the heat setting at all.

3. Mix the mayo with the whipped cream. Mix in your desired spices, continuing to cook it until mayo cooks through. Lower the heat, stirring.

4. Make spirals of the zucchini with a spiralizer. Someone without a spiralizer can make a thin zucchini strip by using a potato peeler.

5. Put the noodles in a bowl and heat them on the highest setting in a microwave for three minutes. Be sure to heat them until they gain a crunchy texture.

6. In another bowl, put the egg yolks together with diced bacon and parmesan.

7. Add the fat from the bacon to the newly made cream sauce and noodles, mixing them until they are totally coated. Make sure the mix is warm. Next, add the egg-

bacon-parmesan mix into the noodles. Mix them all together. When you do this, the egg mix will become scrambled if they are warm enough when you mix them. If that's not what you want, don't let them get too warm.

8. Split across four plates. Finish off with plenty of your parmesan cheese.

Day 5: Keto Bread

I've tried many recipes that claim to be a worthy substitute for wheat bread. This one is my favorite by far. This recipe is definitely going to please your taste buds.

Ingredients:

- 1 and a half cups Almond Flour
- Separate 6 Large eggs into yolks and whites
- Quarter cup melted Butter
- 3 teaspoons Baking Powder
- 1/4 teaspoon Cream of Tartar (optional but puts the texture closer to regular bread)
- 1 pinch of Salt
- Liquid Stevia (optional but I find around 6 drops helps to mask the egg taste)

Directions:

1. Preheat oven to 375°F.

2. Coat an 8x4 loaf pan with butter and set it aside.

3. Beat the egg whites until they begin to take on a creamy look. With optional cream of tartar, it will begin to form peaks similar to the appearance of meringue on a pie when finished. Note: egg whites whip better in a metal or ceramic bowl as opposed to plastic. You may still achieve the peaks without cream of tartar but at the cost of more beating. Set them aside.

4. Use a food processor to blend egg yolks, a third of the whites, butter, flour, baking powder, salt, and the Stevia if you plan to use any. Mix them briefly until you have a thick lumpy dough.

5. Add the remaining egg whites and mix them on a lower setting. It is important to only mix just enough to blend the egg whites into the dough. Too much mixing will eliminate the fluffy texture that we're trying to keep in the bread.

6. Place the dough in the pre-greased baking pan. Bake for 30 minutes. Check the bread with a toothpick and make sure it comes out clean before removing. I usually get about 20 slices out of a loaf, but you can decide your preferred thickness.

Day 6: Keto Pizza

If you haven't tried Fat Head dough yet, it is a great and crispy substitute for pizza dough. This version of pizza has just 3 carbs a slice, making it great for the Keto diet or simply for cutting carbs.

Ingredients:

- 1 1/2 cups Shredded Mozzarella cheese
- 1 egg
- 2 Tablespoons of cream cheese
- Teaspoon of baking powder
- 3/4 cups almond flour
- Desired herbs and spices
- Pizza sauce and Toppings of choice

Directions:

1. Preheat oven to 450°F.

2. Add both cheeses to a bowl and microwave for 40-45 seconds until soft.

   After microwaving, add egg, almond flour, baking powder, and your desired seasoning (I recommend garlic at least). Mix well with a spoon.

3. Parchment paper is essential to prevent this dough from sticking to everything. Lay a piece out flat, place dough on it, and place another piece on top. Flatten the dough with a rolling pin to roughly ¼ inches thick. Remove the top piece of paper and fine-tune the dough with your hands if necessary for a perfect shape.

4. Move the bottom piece of parchment paper onto your baking sheet or pizza stone to transfer the dough. Baking it without the paper underneath will result in a strong bond with your baking pan, so it is not recommended. Bake it for 10 minutes. If you find the crust isn't strong enough, you can flip the crust using parchment paper mid-bake for stronger crust.

5. Once the crust has baked and is ready, pull it from the oven and add your chosen sauce and any meats and veggies.

6. Put the pizza back in the oven for 5-8 more minutes or until your cheese is bubbly.

Day 7: Keto Frittata

Frittatas are a great breakfast all-in-one. Great for the Keto diet and simplifying everything on your plate into one item.

Ingredients:

- Diced bacon or chorizo
- 2 tablespoons butter
- 8 ounces fresh spinach
- 8 eggs
- 1 cup whipping cream (heavy)
- 5 ounces of your preferred shredded cheese
- salt and pepper

Directions:

1. Preheat the oven to 350°F. Coat the 9x9 ceramic baking dish with butter or individual ramekins if you have them.

2. Fry the bacon or chorizo and butter in the skillet on medium. Heat until crispy. Throw in spinach and keep stirring until wilted. Remove from the burner and keep

warm.

3. Whisk the cream and eggs together and pour them into your baking dish, or separate them into ramekins.

4. Top with the mixture from the skillet and place it in the center of the oven. Bake it until the top turns golden brown, which takes about 25 or 30 minutes.

Day 8: Keto BLT

Another breakfast staple is the BLT. It is a convenient sandwich that's so good—people don't just eat it in the mornings! I find that this Cloud Bread recipe makes for a great BLT. It is like taking the egg out of the sandwich and morphing it into the bun. I hope you enjoy it too.

Ingredients:

- Cloud bread
- 3 eggs
- 4 ounces/half package cream cheese
- Pinch salt
- ½ tablespoon ground psyllium husk powder (you can order this online or find it at your local supplement shop. It is a beneficial item to work into your diet)
- ½ teaspoon baking powder
- ¼ teaspoon cream of tartar (optional as before)

Filling:

- Mayonnaise
- Bacon (cooked)
- Lettuce

- Tomato, sliced

Directions:

Bread:

1. Preheat the oven to 300°F.

2. Separate the eggs into yolks and whites.

3. Add the salt and cream of tartar (if you have it) to the egg whites and beat the mixture until you achieve peaks. If you can turn the bowl upside down without losing the egg whites, you're done.

4. In the bowl containing the egg yolks, mix in psyllium husk, cream cheese, and baking powder.

5. Slowly mix in the egg whites using a folding motion, being careful to preserve the fluff of the mixture, as too much mixing will flatten out your bread.

6. On your baking pan covered in parchment paper, scoop the mix into roughly biscuit sized piles and use

a spatula to flatten to about 1/2 inch thick.

7. Bake in the middle of your oven for 25 minutes. They will turn golden brown.

Assembling the BLT:

1. Flip two pieces of the cloud bread; the top during baking will be the outside of the "buns."

2. Spread mayo on each slice.

3. Layer bacon, lettuce, and tomato as desired.

Day 9: Keto Coconut Porridge

For people that typically start their day with oatmeal, I recommend trying this Keto option. It is a healthier alternative with a nice coconut flavor.

Ingredients:

- 1 egg
- 1 tablespoon coconut flour
- Pinch ground psyllium husk powder
- Pinch salt
- 1 ounce butter or coconut oil
- 4 tablespoons coconut cream

Directions:

1. Beat the egg in a small bowl, mix in coconut flour, psyllium husk powder, and salt.

2. In a pan on a low heat setting, melt the butter and coconut cream together. Gently whisk in the egg mixture and mix until it becomes a creamy, thick texture.

3. As with oatmeal, top it with any desired fruits and berries. Instead of adding milk, you can serve with coconut milk or cream.

Day 10: Keto Tex-Mex Casserole

This delicious carb-free casserole is sure to satisfy your craving for a little spice (or a lot if you add more jalapeños). It is a delicious casserole that has the added benefit of making very yummy leftovers.

Ingredients:

- Between 1 and 2 pounds of ground beef
- 1 cup (8 ounces) crushed tomatoes
- 2 tablespoons of butter
- 3 tablespoons your choice of Tex-Mex seasoning
- Pickled jalapeños (1/4 cup recommended, increase for more spice)
- 7 ounces shredded cheese (Monterrey Jack recommended)
- Serve with:
- Sour cream
- Finely chopped scallion/green onion
- Leafy greens or iceberg lettuce
- Guacamole (optional)

Directions:

1. Preheat the oven to 400°F.

2. Fry the ground beef in a skillet with butter on medium-high heat. The beef is done when it has all browned, and there are no traces of pink anywhere.

3. Stir the Tex-Mex seasoning and crushed tomatoes into the skillet with beef. Simmer together for 5 minutes. Taste mixture to determine if you need to add more seasoning or salt and pepper.

4. Pour the contents of the skillet into a 9" baking or casserole dish. Add jalapeños and cheese on top of the beef mixture.

5. Bake the dish in the center of the upper rack of the oven for 15 to 20 minutes. The top will be golden brown.

6. Mix chopped scallions with sour cream in the dish to serve alongside casserole.

7. Add casserole to sour cream mix, lettuce, and guacamole as desired.

Day 11: Chorizo with Creamed Green Cabbage

Spicy chorizo and creamy cabbage make for quite the pair in this dish. The hint of citrus adds a delightful finish, and the lack of carbs makes this dish perfect.

Ingredients:

- Creamed green cabbage
- One small to medium head of green cabbage, roughly 1½ pounds
- 2 tablespoons butter
- 1½ cups whipping cream (heavy)
- Salt and pepper
- ½ cup finely chopped parsley
- ½ tablespoon lemon zest
- Fried chorizo
- 1½ pounds chorizo (you can use regular sausage if you prefer)
- 2 tablespoons butter

Directions:

1. Fry the chorizo with butter in the skillet over medium heat. When it is finished, you'll need to keep it warm until it is ready to serve.

2. Shred the cabbage in a food processor or chop it with a knife.

3. Sauté the cabbage with butter in a skillet over medium heat while stirring on and off until the cabbage is a golden brown. Smaller pieces of cabbage make this much easier if you're chopping it with a knife.

4. Add whipping cream to the sautéed cabbage and heat it to a light boil. Turn the burner to low and let it simmer to reduce cream. (Remember to keep it at the sweet spot below boiling, so you are evaporating as much moisture out as possible while preventing burning or scorching.) Add salt and pepper if you like.

5. Scatter parsley and lemon zest over the cabbage beside the fried chorizo immediately before serving.

Day 12: Keto Mushroom Omelet

The mushroom omelet is a quick and easy dish. If you already have chopped onion and mushrooms, you can assemble this meal anytime in less than ten minutes!

Ingredients:

- 3 eggs
- 1 tablespoon butter
- 1 ounce shredded cheese
- ¼ cup chopped onion (I prefer yellow)
- 4 sliced mushrooms, any variety will do
- salt and pepper

Directions:

1. Mix the eggs in a bowl with a fork until they are smooth in consistency.

2. In a frying pan using medium heat, add butter followed by mushrooms and onion to the pan. They only need to be sautéed long enough to soften. When mushrooms and onions are ready, pour the egg into the skillet.

3. Let the omelet cook until you start to see the sides become solid, indicating that the bottom half is cooking. While the top surface is still liquid, sprinkle the cheese over the omelet.

4. Use a spatula to carefully separate from the pan around the edges of the omelet, then fold half over onto the other half. When the bottom begins to turn golden brown, it is done and ready to slide onto the plate. Sprinkle it with salt and pepper as desired.

Day 13: Keto Lasagna

If you enjoy lasagna, you're sure to enjoy this Keto version. We make our own sheets of Keto pasta that taste just like the real thing.

Ingredients:

Lasagna Sheets:

- 5 tablespoons ground psyllium husk powder
- 8 eggs
- 8-ounce package of cream cheese
- Teaspoon salt

Meat Sauce:

- 2 tablespoons olive oil
- 1 chopped up onion (I recommend yellow)
- 1 chopped up garlic clove
- 1¼ pounds ground beef
- 3 tablespoons tomato paste
- ½ tablespoon basil
- Teaspoon salt

- ¼ teaspoon black pepper
- Half cup water

Cheese Topping:

- 2 cups sour cream (I use crème fraîche instead)
- 5 ounces shredded mozzarella cheese
- 2 ounces grated parmesan cheese
- ½ teaspoon salt
- ¼ teaspoon pepper
- ½ cup fresh parsley

Directions:

Lasagna sheets:

1. Preheat the oven to 300°F.

2. Put the eggs, cream cheese, and salt in a bowl and beat them until they are smooth. Keep beating while you add psyllium husk and set them aside.

3. On a sheet of parchment paper, pour half the mixture and sandwich between paper. Use a rolling pin to flatten it out to roughly 13x18" and transfer the paper with the mixture to the baking sheet. Repeat this with

the remaining half of the mixture. If you are limited to only one oven rack or baking sheet, they can be baked separately.

4. Bake for about 10-12 minutes after removing the top sheet of parchment paper. Set it aside to cool while preparing the rest of the dish. Turn oven up to 400°F for the next step when done baking the pasta.

Meat Sauce:

1. Preheat the skillet with the olive oil over medium-high heat. Put in chopped onion and garlic and sauté until soft. Follow with the beef, tomato paste, and spices. Mix everything together and cook until the beef is done. Cook until the meat is entirely brown with no hint of pink remaining.

2. Pour in water and heat it to a light boil. Reduce the heat and simmer until most of the water has evaporated (it usually takes around 15 minutes). Keep in mind these lasagna sheets are not going to soak up as much water as normal pasta, so we want this sauce to be on the thicker side. Set it aside when enough water has evaporated.

3. Prepare a 9x12" baking dish for the lasagna by lightly greasing.

Cheese Topping:

1. Mix mozzarella cheese and sour cream together. Add parmesan cheese, saving enough to sprinkle on top of the assembled dish for topping. Stir in salt, pepper, and parsley.

2. Before assembling the lasagna, the baked Keto pasta needs to be sliced for layering. I recommend cutting them in half so that you can do a layer in just two pieces. Place pasta sheets in the bottom of the baking dish and cover with half the meat sauce. Cover with the remaining Keto pasta and add the remaining meat sauce.

3. Spread out the cheese mixture on top and sprinkle on the remaining parmesan cheese.

4. Put in the oven at 400°F for about 30 minutes or when the cheese on top has achieved a browned surface. Serve with salad and your choice of dressing.

Day 14: Turkey with Cream Cheese Sauce

This recipe is great on its own, but it also serves as a great starting point. You can mix it up with veggies, cauliflower rice, or quinoa.

Ingredients:

- 2 tablespoons butter
- Turkey breast ~close to 1.5 lbs.
- 2 cups whipping cream (heavy) or crème fraîche
- 8 ounces cream cheese
- A tablespoon soy sauce (I recommend Tamari)
- salt and pepper
- 1 1/4 cup small capers
- Meat thermometer for poultry

Directions:

1. Preheat the oven to 350°F.

2. In an oven-safe frying pan, melt half of the butter over medium heat. Season turkey breasts with salt, pepper, and any other spices you enjoy, and then fry it in the

pan until golden brown.

3. When the outside skin of the turkey breast is golden brown, place the skillet in the oven. Check the turkey breasts with the thermometer every 10 minutes or so until it reaches an internal temperature of at least 165°F. (The time will vary, as larger cuts will take longer than smaller ones.) When the chicken is finished baking, move the turkey breasts to a plate and cover it with a foil tent to retain heat.

4. Pour the juices remaining in the skillet off to a saucepan. Put in whipping cream (or crème fraîche) and cream cheese. Heat it to a light boil while stirring. Then turn the heat to low and let it simmer to thicken the sauce. Add soy sauce and salt and pepper.

5. Melt the rest of the butter in a skillet over high heat and add capers. Sauté the capers until they are crispy. This should not take very long.

6. Serve the turkey with fried capers and pour the sauce on top.

Day 15: Boiled Eggs With Mayo

This is one recipe I always enjoy for those times you don't have time to cook or just don't feel like it. The boiled eggs can be kept in the refrigerator until you want them, so you don't have to eat them right away. You can make them ahead of time and save them for a time you don't want to cook. Pair it with ripe avocado or mayo, and it is a Keto snack.

Ingredients:

- 8 eggs
- Mayonnaise or avocado if desired

Directions:

1. In a pot, bring several inches of water to a steady boil.

2. I use an egg piercer to prevent the eggs from cracking during boiling. If you don't have one, it is not a requirement. Just make sure that if any crack, you eat those first.

3. Place the eggs in the water gently. Make sure there's enough water to cover all the eggs, so they aren't

exposed.

4. Use the guide here to determine how long to boil your eggs if you aren't already used to your own methods. I personally prefer hard-boiled, as I think it is easier to remove the shell, but everyone is different.

    - Soft-boiled   5-6 mins.
    - Medium   6-8 mins.
    - Hard-Boiled 8-10 mins.

5. Serve the eggs plain or with mayonnaise or avocado.

Day 16: Keto Beef Stew

Beef stew is a great hearty meal any time of year, but especially in the colder months. This is one recipe that doesn't need much changing to be Keto-friendly, so you may not even remember you're on a diet with this one!

Ingredients:

- 2 lb. beef roast, cut into pieces no bigger than 1"
- Salt
- Black pepper
- 2 tablespoons olive oil
- 8 ounces sliced mushrooms
- 1 small onion
- 1 large carrot
- 2 stalks celery
- 3 cloves minced garlic
- A tablespoon tomato paste
- Six cups beef broth
- A teaspoon thyme leaves
- 1 teaspoon chopped rosemary

Directions:
1. Peel the carrot and slice it into disks. Chop the onion and celery into small pieces.
2. Preheat a pot on medium heat with olive oil. Pad the beef roast dry with paper towels and season it generously with salt and pepper. Sear beef on all sides until golden brown for no more than a few minutes per side. You will most likely need to repeat this step, as you only want a single layer of beef cuts in the skillet at a time. It won't hurt anything to cook it in batches. Remove from it from the pot when it is finished and add fresh beef until all is cooked. Add additional oil as needed.
3. When you are finished cooking the beef, and it has all been removed from the pan, toss in mushrooms and cook them to light crispy golden, or for about 5 minutes. Add the onion, carrots, and celery and continue cooking for about 5 more minutes. Add the garlic and continue for another minute. Pour in the tomato paste and stir.
4. Add the thyme, broth, rosemary, and beef to the pot. When hot, add salt and pepper to the pot as needed. Briefly boil the stew, then reduce the burner to low and simmer the beef until it is tender. This should take from 50 minutes to an hour.

Day 17: Keto Stuffed Cabbage

The main change with this dish is the replacement of rice with cauliflower rice. You can buy it from the store, but it is fairly easy to make at home. You can make many dishes Keto-friendly by substituting rice with cauliflower rice.

Ingredients:

Sauce:

- 14 ounce can tomatoes diced
- A tablespoon apple cider vinegar
- 1/2 teaspoon red pepper flakes
- A teaspoon onion powder
- A teaspoon garlic powder
- A teaspoon oregano
- Salt
- Black pepper
- Quarter cup olive oil

Cabbage Rolls:

- Cabbage leaves
- 1 lb. ground beef

- 3/4 pound ground pork
- A cup riced cauliflower
- 3 sliced scallions/green onions
- Quarter cup chopped fresh parsley
- Black pepper

Directions:

Sauce:

1. Preheat the oven to 375°F. In a blender, puree tomatoes, apple cider vinegar, pepper flakes, oregano, and onion and garlic powders. Puree the mixture; taste and season it with salt and pepper.

2. Heat the olive oil in a large pot over medium heat. Add the puree sauce from the blender. Bring it to a simmer and hold it for 20 minutes. The sauce will thicken.

Cabbage Rolls:

1. In a pot, boil the water and add the cabbage leaves. Blanch it for about one minute until tender. Set aside.

2. Prepare the filling: in a bowl, mix ½ cup of sauce, meats, cauliflower rice, scallions/green onions, and most of the parsley. Season it with salt and pepper.

3. In the baking dish, spread the first sauce on the bottom. Cut out any rib from each of the cabbage leaves that were too large to soften during blanching. To form cabbage rolls, lay out each leaf and put meat sauce on one end. Roll from the end with sauce and fold the sides in as you roll. Place each roll seam facing down into the baking dish. When all have been formed, gently spoon the remaining sauce over the rolls. Bake from 45 minutes to 55 minutes.

4. Garnish it with remaining parsley to serve.

Day 18: Keto Mac and Cheese

If you like Mac and Cheese, this Keto version is a great substitute. For those that really enjoy the crispy top usually created with bread crumbs, we even have a solution for that.

Ingredients:

Mac and Cheese:

- Butter
- 2 heads cauliflower rinsed and cut into little pieces
- Two tablespoons olive oil
- Salt
- A cup of heavy cream
- Six ounces of cream cheese
- Four cups of shredded cheddar cheese
- Two cups of shredded mozzarella cheese
- Ground black pepper

Topping:

- 4 ounces crushed pork rinds
- 1/4 cup grated Parmesan cheese

- A tablespoon olive oil
- Parsley for garnish

Directions:

1. Preheat the oven to 375°F. Use the butter to grease a 9x13" baking dish. Toss in the cauliflower pieces with the olive oil in a bowl and season it with salt. Spread the cauliflower out onto one (or two if necessary) baking sheets and roast in the oven for about 40 minutes.

2. While the cauliflower is in the oven, heat the cream in a pot on medium heat. Simmer, then turn down the heat to low and stir in the cheeses about a cup at a time until it is all melted. Take it off the burner and season it with salt and pepper (I find that adding a tablespoon of hot sauce provides a nice bit of flavor, but it is entirely optional). Gently fold in the roasted cauliflower.

3. Transfer to a greased baking dish. In a bowl, mix the crushed pork rinds, Parmesan, and 1 tablespoon of olive oil. Sprinkle over the cauliflower and cheese.

4. Bake it for about 15 minutes or to golden brown. Feel free to finish with a couple minutes of the broiler if you really like that crust on top.

5. Garnish with parsley.

Day 19: Keto Fried Chicken

Traditional fried chicken has a few requirements that don't work for the Keto diet, but I bet you won't even notice this isn't fried chicken when you try it. This variation is baked, as it is a much bigger challenge to get the breading to hold up when frying it in a pan as opposed to baking.

Ingredients:

- 6 bone-in, skin-on pieces of chicken
- Salt
- Ground black pepper
- 2 large eggs
- Half cup heavy cream
- 3/4 cup almond flour
- 1.5 cup crushed pork rinds
- Half cup grated Parmesan
- A teaspoon garlic powder
- Half teaspoon paprika
- Spicy Mayo Sauce - Not necessary, but I like to add a couple teaspoons of hot sauce to a 1/2 cup of mayo to pair with this chicken.

Directions:

1. Preheat the oven to 400°F. Put some parchment paper on a baking sheet. Pat the chicken with paper towels and rub it with salt and pepper.

2. Assemble your workspace. You'll want two bowls for dipping next to your baking sheet. In the first bowl, whisk the eggs and heavy cream. In the second, mix the almond flour, pork rinds, Parmesan, garlic powder, and paprika.

3. One-piece at a time, dip or coat the chicken in the first bowl with egg mixture. Then in the dry mix, press to coat it with as much as possible to increase crispness. Finally, place it on the baking sheet.

4. Bake about 45 minutes for breasts, and slightly less for smaller cuts. Chicken should be golden brown outside, and the internal temperature should be at least 165°.

5. The chicken is ready to eat. Don't forget to try it with the homemade spicy mayo.

Day 20: Keto Broccoli Salad

Broccoli salad is a great Keto substitute for pasta salad. I actually prefer it, as the broccoli retains the crunch in the salad, unlike soft pasta. I do recommend making this one ahead of time. While it is good when done, I think it is even better the next day after spending a night in the refrigerator.

Ingredients:

Salad:

- Salt
- 3 heads broccoli cut into small florets
- 1/2 cups shredded Cheddar
- Quarter onion, thinly sliced (Red is preferred for salad, but Vidalia are great too)
- 1/4 cup toasted sliced almonds
- 1/3 cup bacon pieces
- 2 tablespoons chopped chives

Dressing:

- 2/3 cup mayonnaise
- Three tablespoons of apple cider vinegar

- A tablespoon Dijon mustard
- Salt
- Ground black pepper

Directions:

1. In a pot, boil 6 cups of salted water. A similar-sized pot or bowl should be nearby containing ice water.

2. Dump the broccoli florets into the boiling water and cook them for 2 minutes. With a strainer or slotted spoon, fish the broccoli from the boiling water and place it in the ice water. Once they are cool, drain the florets in a colander and allow them to continue draining while making the dressing.

3. Mix all the dressing ingredients in a bowl and taste it, adding salt and pepper as needed.

4. Mix the broccoli with the remaining salad ingredients and dressing. Mix them until it is evenly coated. Eat it or put it in the refrigerator until serving.

Day 21: Keto Meatballs

These meatballs are definitely an improvement over traditional ones made with flour. Quick and easy assembly allows for more time to make a Keto dessert or side.

Ingredients:

Meatballs:
- 1 lb. ground beef
- A clove minced garlic
- Half cup shredded mozzarella
- Grated parmesan
- Two tablespoons chopped fresh parsley
- A large egg
- A teaspoon salt
- Half teaspoon black pepper
- 2 tablespoons olive oil

Sauce:
- 1 chopped onion
- 2 cloves minced garlic
- 28 ounce can crushed tomatoes
- A teaspoon of dried oregano
- Salt
- Black pepper

Directions:

1. For the meatballs, place a skillet with olive oil over medium heat. In a bowl, mix all the remaining meatball ingredients together thoroughly. Form them into 16 meatballs.

2. Add the meatballs to the skillet and turn them occasionally for about 10 minutes. The meatballs should appear golden brown on all sides. Cover a plate with several layers of paper towels. As the meatballs are finished cooking, place them on paper towels to wait.

3. Once all the meatballs are finished cooking and removed from skillet, add onion and cook them for a few minutes to soften. Add garlic and continue for one minute. Add tomatoes and oregano. Taste the sauce and use salt and pepper if necessary.

4. Return the meatballs to the skillet and roll through the sauce. Cover the skillet and simmer for about 15 minutes until the sauce has thickened. Sprinkle with Parmesan when serving.

Day 22: Keto Garlic Rosemary Pork Chops

Pork chops can be quite mouthwatering when done right. The main problem people have with them is making them too dry or too tough, but this recipe is designed for you to enjoy them without running into either problem.

Ingredients:

- 4 pork chops
- Salt
- Black pepper
- A tablespoon rosemary
- 2 cloves minced garlic
- Half cup melted butter
- 1 tablespoon olive oil

Directions:

1. Preheat the oven to 375°F and sprinkle the pork chops with pepper and salt.

2. Mix rosemary and garlic into the melted butter and set them aside.

3. Preheat the olive oil over the burner on medium-high heat in an oven-safe skillet able to accommodate all 4 cuts simultaneously. Sear the pork chops until golden for about 4 minutes on each side.

4. Brush the pork chops with some of the butter mixture and place the skillet in the oven. Bake for about 12 minutes. Keep a 145°F internal temperature, using the thermometer to measure. Serve them with more garlic butter.

Day 23: Keto Cheesy Bacon Ranch Chicken

This recipe for cheesy chicken breast is quite a treat for something so simple. While the ranch seasoning part is optional, you won't want to leave that ingredient out if you enjoy ranch dressing.

Ingredients:

- 4 thick bacon slices
- Four boneless skinless chicken breasts
- Salt
- Black pepper
- Two tsp. ranch seasoning
- 1 and 1/2 cups shredded mozzarella cheese
- Chopped chives

Directions:

1. In a skillet large enough to accommodate all the chicken breasts simultaneously, cook the bacon over medium heat. When you are finished, place the bacon on paper towels to absorb the grease. Depending on how fatty the bacon was, you may have to drain some

fat. You want no more than a couple tablespoons left in the skillet.

2. Season the chicken with salt and pepper and add it to the skillet with bacon grease. Turn up the stove to medium-high heat. Cook the chicken until it is golden brown on all sides.

3. Reduce the heat to medium. If you are using ranch seasoning, sprinkle it over the chicken in the skillet first. Then follow with mozzarella cheese. Cover the pan and continue cooking for about 5 minutes longer.

4. Serve with the bacon pieces and chives on top.

Day 24: Keto Bacon Sushi

Being on a Keto diet can make it seem like you have fewer snack options. This recipe is great because it gives you a new snack option that you wouldn't have tried before you went Keto. If you like sushi, you know how flexible it is in terms of ingredients. Aside from the bacon and cream cheese, you can substitute in whatever veggies you like here.

Ingredients:

- Bacon slices cut in half, each slice will make two pieces
- Cucumber
- Carrot
- Avocado
- 4 ounces softened cream cheese
- Sesame seeds (optional)

Directions:

1. Preheat the oven to 400°F. To prepare the bacon in the oven with minimal cleanup, we will need to take aluminum foil and form it into a baking sheet with sides to catch drippings. Place the bacon on a cooling rack on the foil to suspend it above the pan while cooking, but allowing grease to drip off. Bake it for 11-

13 minutes, as it should be slightly crisp, but still pliable to roll into sushi.

2. Cut the cucumbers, carrots, and avocado into small stick-like pieces. You want them to be about the width of a strip of bacon lengthwise, but it doesn't need to be precise, as this won't affect the taste.

3. When the bacon is cooled enough to touch, spread a thin layer of cream cheese on top of each slice. Place your desired mix of vegetables for each piece of sushi on one end of the bacon and roll the piece up tightly.

4. Your Keto sushi is now ready! For appearance, you can sprinkle on the sesame seeds.

Day 25: Keto Taco Casserole

This taco casserole is so good, you'll be saying "No hablo carbohydrates." Add in chili powder or extra jalapeños for extra spice.

Ingredients:

- A tablespoon of olive oil
- Half diced onion (Yellow recommended)
- 2 pounds ground beef
- 2 tablespoons salt
- Ground black pepper
- 2 tablespoons Keto-friendly (no added sugars) taco seasoning mix
- One minimum jalapeño, seeded and finely chopped, slices for garnish
- 6 large eggs
- 2 cups shredded cheese (Monterrey Jack recommended or a taco cheese blend)
- 2 tablespoons chopped parsley
- Serve with sour cream (optional)

Directions:

1. Preheat the oven to 350°F. Place the olive oil in the skillet on medium heat. Dump in the chopped onion and sauté until it is gold and softened.

2. Cook the ground beef, salt, and pepper. Cook the beef until brown and there is no pink. Break up the beef into the desired size of pieces while cooking. Mix the taco seasoning and chopped jalapeño. When the seasoning has blended into the beef after a minute or two, drain the grease from the pan and keep it warm.

3. Whisk the eggs in a bowl, then mix in the meat mixture. In a baking dish (2 quarts or larger), place the mixture in the bottom. Then cover it with the cheese. You can also add jalapeños on top of the cheese if you like.

4. Bake for 25 minutes.

5. Garnish with parsley. Serve with additional jalapeño slices and sour cream if desired.

Day 26: Keto Chicken Parmesan

If you don't enjoy chicken Parmesan, then you either have not tasted the right dish or don't like chicken. I think this one tastes better than what you get at certain popular restaurants.

Ingredients:

- Four boneless, skinless chicken breasts
- Salt
- Black pepper
- One cup almond flour
- Three large eggs
- 3 cups grated Parmesan
- Two tsps. garlic powder
- One tsp. onion powder
- Two tsps. oregano
- Two tbsp. Vegetable oil
- Three quarter cup tomato sauce (if you can't find one without added sugar try pureed tomatoes)
- 1 1/2 cups shredded mozzarella
- Garnish with basil leaves

Directions:

1. Preheat the oven to 400°F and slice the chicken in half crosswise, so they are the same size, just half as thick. Season the chicken with salt and pepper.

2. For the breading setup, we need three bowls. In the first bowl, put in the almond flour. In the second bowl, beat the eggs. In the third bowl, mix Parmesan, garlic and onion powders, and oregano with a little bit of salt and pepper.

3. Dip the chicken cutlets into the almond flour first, then the eggs, and then Parmesan mixture. Press just like you were making fried chicken.

4. Add vegetable oil to a large skillet and preheat on medium heat. Put in the chicken and cook it for about 3 minutes on each side. If not all the chicken fits in the skillet together, just cook it in batches, making sure to add more oil if needed.

5. Place the cutlets in a 9x13" baking dish after the skillet. Pour some tomato sauce over each cutlet and sprinkle it with cheese.

6. Put in the oven for 10-12 minutes until the cheese melts. Browning can be achieved with broiler if desired.

7. Sprinkle with Parmesan and garnish with a basil leaf to serve.

Day 27: Keto Meatloaf

This is not your grandmother's meatloaf. This is a decidedly new twist on a classic with some impressive flavor. It is everything you love about meatloaf and then some!

Ingredients:

- Cooking spray
- One tbsp. olive oil
- One onion (yellow recommended)
- 1 stalk celery
- 3 cloves minced garlic
- One tsp oregano
- One tsp chili powder
- 2 pounds ground beef
- One cup shredded cheddar cheese
- Half cup almond flour
- Quarter cup grated Parmesan cheese
- 2 eggs
- 1 tablespoon soy sauce (I still recommend Tamari)
- Salt

- Black pepper
- 6 bacon strips

Directions:

1. Preheat the oven to 400°F. Rinse and chop the onion and celery. Coat a baking dish with the cooking spray. Put the olive oil in a skillet on medium heat. Sauté the onion and celery for several minutes, then put in garlic, oregano, and chili powder. Cook for another minute, then remove from heat.

2. Mix the beef, the contents of the skillet, and the remainder of the ingredients except bacon together in a bowl. Add salt and pepper. Shape the mixture and place it in the baking dish, then drape the bacon slices over the meatloaf. You'll want to make sure the bacon is pressed against the meatloaf, as space between may result in the bacon cooking too fast. If this happens, you can create a foil tent for the dish to slow down the bacon cook speed.

3. Bake for 1 hour.

Day 28: Keto Garlicky Lemon Mahi-Mahi

There isn't much you have to change about a fish filet to make it Keto-friendly. In fact, this one is a pretty standard recipe that's tried, true, and already Ketogenic.

Ingredients:

- 2 tablespoons olive oil
- Three tablespoons butter
- Four small mahi-mahi fillets
- Salt
- Ground black pepper
- 1 pound asparagus
- Three cloves minced garlic
- Quarter tsp. crushed red pepper flakes
- 1 lemon
- Fresh parsley

Directions:

1. Using a grater, zest the lemon into a bowl. Remember, you only want the yellow of the skin, not the white underneath. Then halve the lemon and squeeze out the

juice into the zest. Discard the remaining lemon and set the bowl aside for later.

2. Add 1 tbsp of olive oil and 1 tbsp of butter to a skillet on medium heat. When hot, put in the fish and season it with some pepper and salt. Cook for four or five minutes per side until it golden brown, then place on a plate.

3. Using the rest of the olive oil with asparagus, add it to the skillet and cook it until it is tender. Add pepper and salt and move it to the second plate.

4. Place the rest of the butter in the skillet and sauté the garlic and red pepper flakes for one minute. Then stir in the bowl of lemon juice and zest with a bit of chopped parsley. Remove the skillet from the heat and return the mahi-mahi and asparagus to the skillet. Pour sauce over them.

5. Serve garnished with a sprig of parsley.

Day 29: Keto Philly Cheesesteak Lettuce Wraps

This version of Keto-friendly cheesesteak is a treasure. Is it authentic? Of course not, but unless you're a Philadelphia cheesesteak purist, you don't care as long as it tastes good. If you have any Chicago native friends, entertain them by putting ketchup on your hot dog.

Ingredients:

- 2 tablespoons vegetable oil
- One big onion
- Two big bell peppers
- One teaspoon oregano
- Salt
- Black pepper
- One lb. skirt steak
- One cup shredded provolone cheese
- Butterhead lettuce leaves
- Fresh Parsley

Directions:

1. Rinse the vegetables and slice the onion, bell peppers, and steak.

2. Preheat one tablespoon of vegetable oil in the skillet on medium heat. Sauté onion and bell peppers until tender with oregano, pepper, and salt. Remove and keep peppers and onions warm. Then add the remaining oil to skillet.

3. Add the steak to the skillet and sprinkle pepper and salt to season. Cook it for about two minutes to sear the steak, then flip and cook the steak to preferred doneness. Another two minutes will be about medium.

4. When the steak is ready, return the vegetables back to the skillet and toss them together. Sprinkle provolone over the mixture and cover the skillet with a lid. Cook it for another minute. Remove from the heat.

5. Arrange the leaves of lettuce on a serving dish or plate. The cheesesteak mixture is served on the lettuce leaves. For extra stability, you may want to use more than one leaf for each. Garnish with parsley.

Day 30: Keto Tuscan Butter Shrimp

This creamy shrimp dish is quite flavorful. The sauce is so good, and this recipe can be used for salmon filets as well instead of being limited to shrimp.

Ingredients:

- Two tbsps. olive oil
- One pound shrimp (assuming these are already prepared, if you buy whole shrimp you'll need to peel and devein them yourself)
- Salt
- Black pepper
- Three tbsps. butter
- Three cloves minced garlic
- One and a half cups cherry tomatoes sliced in half lengthwise
- 3 cups baby spinach
- Half cup heavy cream
- Quarter cup grated Parmesan
- Quarter cup fresh or 2 tablespoons dried basil
- Lemon wedges to garnish (optional)

Directions:

1. Preheat the large skillet with olive oil over medium-high heat. Pepper and salt the shrimp and add the shrimp to the skillet when it is hot. Sear the underside fit about two minutes until golden, and then flip and finish. The shrimp should appear somewhat translucent when it is fully cooked. Remove the shrimp from the skillet and keep warm.

2. Turn down the heat to medium and throw in the butter to melt. Sauté the garlic for one minute and then put in cherry tomatoes with some pepper and salt. Sauté until you see tomatoes begin to burst. Dump in the spinach and continue cooking until the spinach is beginning to wilt.

3. Add cream, Parmesan cheese, and basil and stir. Bring the sauce to a simmer, then turn the heat down and continue at a light simmer until the sauce reduces—about 3-4 minutes.

4. Add the shrimp back to the skillet and stir it. Cook it for 5 minutes to finish. If you are using fresh basil, garnish with a basil leaf and squeeze a bit of lemon juice on top.

Chapter 4: Hormone and Diabetes Support on Keto

Keto works differently for people with Type 2 diabetes. Keto might seem like an odd diet for people with diabetes since a Keto diet is high in fat. However, Keto also causes your body to need less insulin while it simultaneously helps you achieve a healthier blood sugar level.

Since many people with Type 2 diabetes are obese or overweight, a high-fat diet doesn't immediately seem like a good idea. However, this viewpoint is only the result of some misconceptions about Keto and weight gain in general.

People tend to see fat consumption as the main reason for weight gain, but the truth is, people mainly gain weight because they eat high-calorie foods without doing any physical activity to offset it.

Keto shifts the way your body processes energy, and this is easily the biggest change that Keto brings to your body. Whether you are diabetic or not, Keto gives you an entirely new source of energy by way of fats. Keto helps women with diabetes experience fewer of the disease's negative symptoms because their system stops relying on sugar for energy.

Diabetes patients do need to tread more carefully when doing Keto. After all, some women will use Keto as an excuse to eat a lot of high-calorie foods without exercising—as I have said, this is a misguided approach to Keto. Women with diabetes reduce the amount of sugar in their blood by introducing less of it in the first place; most of your sugars probably come from carbs before you do Keto, so cutting carbs means cutting those natural sugars.

When you reduce your body's reliance on sugar for energy, it mitigates the vicious cycle of obesity. I am referring to the cycle in which you constantly introduce new sugar into your bloodstream through carbs. Women with diabetes need less insulin when they do Keto because the diet keeps their blood sugar under control.

With all that said, you should still be aware of the risks associated with tackling diabetes with Keto. First off, some women hear they can eat high-fat foods as long as they reduce their carb intake, and they take this to mean they can eat any foods high in any kind of fat. This is not true. You must specifically eat foods high in unsaturated fats. It is likely the foods you ate before Keto are high in unsaturated fats: foods like beef, pork, and dairy products.

These foods do not have the unsaturated fats we are talking about. The foods rich in unsaturated fats include avocado, vegetable oil, peanut butter, fatty fish, nuts, cashews, and seeds. When you do Keto, you need to stop eating those foods loaded with saturated fats and eat these foods rich in unsaturated fats. Women with diabetes particularly need to watch out for foods high in saturated fats because they can have a grave impact on your body.

Diabetic women who were not on the Keto diet were already following a diet with some of Keto's characteristics. Doctors recommend that diabetic women do not consume many carbohydrates because they increase your blood sugar dramatically compared to other nutrients. When you eat a meal high in carbs, it could cause a rapid increase in blood sugar that is dangerous for people with diabetes.

At the same time, reducing your calorie consumption as a whole is not necessarily healthy either. Your body still needs energy to survive. That's why following Keto is a good idea if you are a woman with diabetes—because you can get your energy from healthy fats instead of carbs.

The most important thing to remember when you do Keto on diabetes is to monitor the level of Ketones in your system. If your Ketones reach a certain threshold—240 mg/dL on your blood sugar tester—this puts you at high risk for diabetic Ketoacidosis (DKA).

It is a much higher risk if you have type 1 diabetes, but if your Ketones are especially high, you are at risk if you have type 2 diabetes as well. No matter what, try to keep your Ketones below this threshold.

Another important recommendation is to keep your doctor updated about your eating habits, especially if you are going all out with Keto. Your doctor will know best what you should eat and how far you should go with Keto.

Recently, there has been a great deal of research on women with diabetes who do Keto. The results have been telling about the wonders it can do for them.

Women who had diabetes and followed the Keto diet for twenty-four weeks had better glycemic control. They also did not need to take as many prescription drugs while they were on the diet. In addition, these women saw the same weight loss that has been seen in research about non-diabetic women doing Keto.

A 2013 metastudy on women with diabetes saw that Keto helps women control their blood sugar, weight, and need for insulin. Women who did not follow Keto and women who did other diets did not see these same benefits.

A 2017 study compared Keto to traditional diets that cut down on fat instead of carbs. Women who did Keto for 32 weeks instead of these other diets had fewer diabetic symptoms and lost more weight.

It is no surprise that Keto is becoming more popular among women with diabetes, and scientists are growing more interested in studying it. Women themselves are seeing how it makes their lives better. If you have diabetes, you can join them to see these results for yourself.

Even if you don't have diabetes, you may be curious about how the Ketogenic diet could influence your hormones. It is an understandable concern, as any diet can change the balance of your hormones. As a woman, it is smart to understand how the food you eat affects the delicate balance of chemicals in your body.

Firstly, know that lowering your carbohydrate consumption induces stress on your body in the beginning. Carbs are difficult for your body to digest, and they contain a lot of glucose, which can have unhealthy consequences. But carbs are also where many people, especially women, get nutrients such as fiber and other vitamins. Besides giving us these vital nutrients, carbs are an integral part of keeping your hormones in balance.

There are three major changes that happen in a woman's hormones when she starts consuming fewer carbs. First, her level of serotonin changes. Insulin metabolism and progesterone also change as a result of lower carb intake.

Know that hormones affect everything that happens in your body, so while you may be most concerned about how hormone changes affect you subjectively, you should also be aware of the great physical impact hormones have on your body.

Hormone levels themselves can have a dramatic effect on a woman's weight. If your hormones change too much and too quickly, this can make us put on weight because of the increase in insulin that often accompanies a change in hormones.

You may be concerned about the potential risk for weight gain that can come with a shift in hormones. This concern may even make you wonder whether you should be doing Keto in the first place.

But you need to consider this fact in its context. Remember that hormone changes are natural and happen all the time, whether we experience a change in diet or not. That means any weight gain you might experience from hormone changes will probably be temporary.

After your body adjusts to the hormonal changes from the lower carb content of your diet, you will start noticing weight loss along with the other positive health effects from Keto.

There are other hormonal factors you might want to consider with Keto as well. Hormonal changes can also have an impact on your levels of cortisol. You might not know what cortisol is, but you certainly know the subjective feeling that comes with it: stress.

Cortisol is the hormone that is flowing through our bodies when we are feeling stressed. In Keto, your cortisol level changes do not usually result from the lowered carb intake itself. Instead, you might feel temporarily stressed because of the "unintended consequences" that can come with low carb intake.

Specific fruits and vegetables should not be consumed when you do Keto because of their starchiness and high carb content. The bad part is, these fruits and vegetables also contain important nutrients. When you do Keto and don't get these foods anymore, you don't get these nutrients. A woman's body can start to produce more cortisol when it doesn't get enough of that nutrient. She starts to feel more stressed as a result.

For example, Keto experts recommend not consuming certain vegetables—usually non-green vegetables—because they are too starchy. Likewise, they tell women not to eat fruit.

But there is a simple solution to this hormonal problem. While you eat Keto-friendly foods, be sure you are still getting the vitamins and minerals your body needs. You won't be able to get them from the same sources as you used to, but you can still get these nutrients in your Ketogenic diet. These include all the vitamins, iron, fiber, calcium, and so forth. You still need to get these nutrients while you are on Keto.

You can still get these nutrients on the Keto diet. The problem is, many women are used to getting them from certain sources that they are no longer supposed to eat while on Keto. You will have to be proactive about getting these nutrients from new sources.

Adjusting to Keto can be hard, whether you are diabetic or not. Women with diabetes have to grapple with all kinds of things that women without it don't, but even if you don't have diabetes, you still need to keep your hormones in check.

In the next chapter, we take a broader look at Keto and give you advice on following it for all kinds of different situations. If you want to know how to make it easier to do Keto by properly managing the ingredients in your kitchen, please read on.

Chapter 5: Keto Tips and Tricks

This chapter is filled with useful tips to keep you on track with Keto. Some of them are relatively simple, while others will help you see things in a new and helpful way. You already know that the essential part of Keto is limiting your carb intake, but that doesn't make it easy to do in practice. This chapter gives you a list of tips that will make it easy.

Our first tip is about shopping for food. If you go grocery shopping with a predetermined list of items based on our 30-day diet plan, you won't even feel the need to buy anything that might contain carbs. You already know that you're buying good foods that stay within the confines of Keto, so it won't even cross your mind.

This tip goes with the most important advice I have for you, which is not to overwhelm yourself.

Overwhelming yourself with all the possibilities of Keto is easy to do. The best way to avoid this is to know the ingredients you need for your meals before you cook them.

You already have a list of 30 meals that all follow the Keto diet's requirements. What comes next is being ready to cook these meals every day. Getting the ingredients in your pantry or fridge is the first thing you need to do.

You don't want to plan to eat the Keto taco casserole the next day and find out you are missing ground beef the day of. You can avoid making this mistake by looking at the ingredient lists ahead of time. Double-check it to make sure you have everything you need ahead of time.

But you might find that keeping track of every ingredient ahead of time is unrealistic. Luckily, there is an easier way to look at these ingredients. You can break down the ingredients you need into three groups: proteins, vegetables, and healthy fats.

The first one is the easiest to find. Be sure you always have protein sources in your home such as turkey, fish, pork, beef, and so on.

When you check your kitchen for vegetables, you want to stick with vegetables that are low in carbs, of course. Examples of vegetables that fit into this category include broccoli, cauliflower, cucumbers, and bell peppers.

Finally, you want to have fats in your diet, but they need to be healthy fats. If you don't know the difference, here is a quick run-down.

We have three basic kinds of fats: from least healthy to healthiest, we have trans fats, saturated fats, and unsaturated fats.

You never want to eat trans fats. In fact, they are even banned in the United States and many other countries. Saturated fats are not good for you, either, but you don't need to be concerned about getting a few grams of saturated fats here and there.

However, you want most of your fats to be unsaturated fats. Unsaturated fats fall into two categories that you will see on nutrition labels: polyunsaturated and monounsaturated fats. Be on the lookout for these, because they are the kinds of fats you want when you are on the Keto diet.

As long as you get unsaturated fats, proteins, and low-carb vegetables into your diet, you are on Keto. The 30 days of recipes will be of great help to you, but you don't need to follow them exactly. You will still be doing Keto if you follow these basic guidelines.

My next tip is to make it impossible to betray your new Keto diet. Women new to the diet often can't get started with it simply because they keep the same food in their house. It is certainly harder to change your diet when all the old foods you used to eat are lying around.

We say to ourselves that we don't want to waste food. Not wanting to waste food is a good virtue, but in practice, it only keeps us from changing our eating habits. We tell ourselves that we can change our habits later, but later never comes.

The only way to keep yourself from making this mistake is to get rid of the risk entirely. As long as you still have high-carb foods in your pantry and refrigerator, there is a very good chance you will still eat them.

I don't like to waste food either, so when I started Keto, I gave these foods to my parents. That way, the food didn't go to waste, but I didn't have to eat it and mess up my Keto routine.

Since you are new to Keto, you might not know what exactly you should get rid of. Now, you still have to make choices every day not to break with Keto. This tip will not keep you from ever "cheating" on Keto—but it will make it a whole lot easier if you give away all these items in your kitchen:

- Grains such as pasta, wheat, bread, rice, and cereal.
- Sweets— anything manufactured to be filled with sugar. This means candy, honey, soda, juice, syrup, chocolate, and cake.
- Potatoes and other starchy vegetables
- Legumes such as beans
- Fruits like oranges, grapes, apples, and bananas that are high in sugar

- Dairy products (they can be consumed in moderation, but you need to seriously limit your consumption of them)
- Processed foods in general. If you have any foods in your kitchen that are less than fresh, you will know what they are. Take these out of your kitchen.

When you rid your kitchen of these foods, you need foods to replace them with. Here is a place to start:

- Butter and coconut oil for their unsaturated fats
- Green vegetables such as kale, spinach, and lettuce
- Any vegetables low in carbohydrates such as cauliflower, asparagus, and zucchini
- Beef, pork, chicken, turkey, fish—any meat really, as long as you get them from a grocery store whose meat sources are grass-fed
- Lots of eggs

My next tip is to know the Keto staples.

In case you don't already know, Keto staples are foods that Keto practitioners eat every single day. Like all Keto foods, they are low-carb and often high in unsaturated fats. These foods are also easy to eat and usually are consumed in the form of snacks. Start replacing high-carb, heavily processed snacks with these Keto staples:

- Seeds and nuts like sunflower seeds, almonds, cashews, and peanuts in small amounts
- Flour substitutes such as coconuts flour and almond flour
- Sweet but sugarless drinks like black coffee and tea. Find a source of sweetening that has no sugar if you don't want to consume them plain
- By the same token, find a sugarless sweetener to give your water some taste

I can't overstate the importance of finding a sugar-free source of sweetener. People who can't stick with Keto sometimes have issues doing so because they feel like they can't get enough flavor while on the diet.

As you know from the 30-day Keto meal plan, this is not true—you can get all kinds of flavors while still on the diet.

The real problem is that people these days have a sugar addiction. We are so used to eating sugar all the time that we feel like we need it. We could criticize ourselves endlessly for being used to eating sweet food, but that wouldn't get us anywhere.

What we really need is a solution to this addiction to sweetness. Since we can't consume too much sugar on Keto, our best option is to replace it with sugarless sweeteners.

Now that we have spent plenty of time helping you to change the foods you eat, we are getting into the psychological side of changing your diet. This next tip is simple: take it easy.

There is a lot of incentive not to jump into Keto without caution. The Keto flu may be only temporary, but it tends to discourage women from continuing to do Keto, so it is still something worth avoiding. You are better off taking things slowly, so you don't shake the balance of your body's chemicals too much.

But how do you actually take it slowly? If you take Keto slowly, where do you start?

The trick to taking Keto slowly is to introduce one new lifestyle change at a time. For example, you could first try taking out all the sugar-filled foods in your kitchen, but don't do anything else. Just see how well you can get by without these foods.

Once you get used to your life without these foods, try to do something else, like eating more vegetables such as broccoli, cauliflower, and spinach. You might be hesitant to take Keto one thing at a time because you want to get the most possible health effect from it as quickly as possible.

However, the risk of burning out of Keto is real. That's why I suggest you make one small change towards Keto at a time—it is much more sustainable in the long term.

In the same vein, pay attention to the signs your body is giving you. You will be able to tell whether you are taking things too quickly or not.

A lot of people go wrong in this area because they get busy with day-to-day life and stop listening to their bodies.

Don't let this happen to you. Allow some time to yourself every day where you aren't consuming any media, whether it is music, TV, or Internet. Do nothing but spend a little bit of time in silence every day.

It doesn't have to be more than five to ten minutes every hour. After that, you can go back to whatever it is you were doing. But especially when you are making such a drastic change to your body, you can't implement all these changes without listening to your body's response to it. Be sure you are ready for your body to tell you what to do next.

Another aspect of improving at listening to your body is realizing how slow your body is to tell you things. A good example of this is how long it takes for it to tell you that you are full.

All of us have experienced this. We finish our dinner, but afterwards, we still feel hungry. Then, we feel justified in continuing to eat because we think our bodies are telling us to keep eating. Even if we know logically that we shouldn't eat anymore, we look for any excuse to just do whatever it is we want to do.

There is a way to deal with this problem.

If you know that you have eaten plenty, but your body is telling you to eat more, find something else to get your mind occupied with for a while. You might still feel hungry after this time, and if so, you should be fine to eat.

That might mean your body really did need more energy. But more likely than not, your body was telling you to eat more because you were bored—or just because it tastes good. People easily confuse genuine hunger with mere craving. You can entertain yourself in ways other than eating so as to avoid this confusion.

My last tip for succeeding in Keto is to know how to approach these three nutrients: carbs, proteins, and healthy fats.

For carbs, you could know nothing more than not to eat more than 30 grams of carbs every day. For protein, try to get 0.9 grams of protein for every pound you weigh. Finally, for fats, try to reach 100 grams of healthy fats every day.

Don't buy into the old paradigm that fats are bad. Fats are not the enemy—the enemy is eating too many calories without burning them off with exercise. Keeping carbs off is the best way to stay away from these extra calories in the first place.

Chapter 6:
How to Reset your Metabolism

Science supports the idea of "set weight." That is, people have different body types—with some people naturally keeping a slimmer figure and others having curvier shape.

With that said, the "set weight" hypothesis doesn't excuse us from living healthily. Of all the health metrics, weight predicts our overall health the most.

That means staying at a healthy weight is the best thing you can do for your health, whether you have a low "set weight" or not. This chapter tells you how to make this happen by resetting your metabolism through Keto.

Resetting your metabolism relies on a biological process that I mentioned in the beginning of the book: autophagy.

As I said then, autophagy and Keto go hand and hand. This chapter tells you how to use Keto and autophagy together to reset your metabolism. That way, you can burn through fat almost as quickly as you did when you were younger.

At the end of the day, the power of autophagy comes from the way it strengthens and enlivens your cells. Without your cells, you wouldn't be able to do anything.

They can be easy to disregard because you can't see them, but the fact is, keeping your cells healthy is the best way you can get your metabolism to where you want it to be.

When we age, our cells don't do their jobs as well as they used to. They undergo wear and tear over time. The process of autophagy is meant to repair this damage, but most people don't go through enough advanced autophagy to repair this damage.

That's because advanced autophagy requires us to stop giving our bodies food. This day in age, it is rare for someone in the developed world to go a day without eating. But this comes at a cost. If we fast, our cells get nutrients from existing sources like damaged organelles proteins and foreign toxins. If we don't fast, the damage from all this cellular waste piles up, causing more wear and tear.

There is no need to fret if you rarely go a day without eating now. You can start combining your Keto diet with autophagy today and help your cells repair from the damage they have undergone over time.

We should be highly motivated to do this because having healthier cells means having better skin, gaining more energy, and of course, having a faster metabolism. Most women who follow the Keto diet are mainly interested in losing weight, but I'm sure you don't mind having these benefits alongside a reset metabolism.

When you don't go through enough autophagy, you gain weight more easily. On the flip side, you have a much easier time losing weight when you give your cells the time to detoxify themselves.

We can break down the word "autophagy" to get a fundamental understanding of what it does. As you likely know, "auto" means self. "Phagy" means eat. Autophagy is when your cell eats itself because you are fasting. Your cells undergo autophagy when you fast because you are not giving them any food from the outside, so they have to get energy by burning dead organelles, proteins, and foreign toxins.

You might need a more specific example of how autophagy affects you in real life. Look no further than the mitochondria.

The mitochondria is the most vital organelle in each of your cells. But your cells can only get rid of damaged mitochondria through autophagy. Without advanced autophagy, your cells' mitochondria will just keep functioning worse than they should.

Your mitochondria are where all of your cells get energy—on the broader scale; your mitochondria are where you get all of your energy in total. When you clean out your damaged mitochondria and replace them with new mitochondria organelles through autophagy, you are able to reset your metabolism. You feel like you have as much energy as when you were young.

To help you get to the point where you can enjoy this enhanced metabolism, I am going to provide you with a guide to the different stages of Keto.

First, we have ten hours after you start Keto. You may only be at the very beginning of the Ketosis and autophagy, but you will notice changes even this early on.

Women report losing some pounds even this early on. This happens even without exercise because your system has to burn through fat for energy when you aren't providing it with carbs to burn glucose. A lot of the fats that are broken down are changed to Ketones, which help you burn fat even more.

It may shock you that you are already burning fat for energy just ten hours in, but the fact is, Ketosis is a process that can get started and stopped extremely quickly.

You are probably excited about how fast these changes occur, but the important thing is to keep up the behaviors that lead to the fat burn. Do not give up when it gets tough—that means you are getting close to seeing results.

Now, we get to the part where your metabolism is improved from Keto. You will already be able to eat more without gaining as much weight.

The reason for this is that autophagy is improved when you are in Ketosis. Since your system is using Ketones for energy instead of glucose, it is easier for your body to maintain advanced autophagy.

You see, when you put sugar-rich nutrients like carbs into your body, this halts advanced autophagy completely. You are giving your cells plenty of outside food to use for energy, so there is no reason for your cells to engage in self-eating.

But when your body is using Ketones for energy instead of glucose, you don't have this problem. Your autophagy will be enhanced, allowing your metabolism to reset.

Women even say they feel psychologically better when they are going through Ketosis. Your brain is depending on Ketones for all its energy, too, leading to a distinct feeling of lucidity.

Now let's skip to 16 hours into Ketosis. Assuming you haven't gotten into Keto before, this is probably the most your body has ever burned through fat before. Be aware that it can lead to some very real physical sensations because of the drastic changes in your body chemistry.

When you are at this stage of Ketosis, you have a tremendous amount of Ketones in your body. It might feel a little physically uncomfortable to drop so much weight at once, so be ready to feel a little sick

At this stage, you might think you did something wrong by doing Keto. But if you know ahead of time that some discomfort is normal, you will be better prepared. It will be obvious if you are actually sick.

One day into the Ketogenic diet, your Ketosis and autophagy are both near the most advanced stages they can be in. The scientific research on autophagy has found that the most advanced level of autophagy you can achieve is after 36 hours into fasting.

This was measured by looking at the number of autophagosomes in the blood; autophagosomes are the specialized vesicles your cells use in autophagy. The more autophagosomes in your blood, the more advanced your autophagy is. After fasting for 36 hours, you have reached the most advanced autophagy you can get.

At this stage in Ketosis, your cells are doing a great job of breaking down cellular waste. After breaking down toxins, your cells turn them into raw material that can be reused to make new organelles and proteins.

Two days into Ketosis, the delicate balance of chemicals and biological mechanisms in your body continues to improve your metabolism. While Ketosis reaches its pinnacle at around 24 hours, the Ketones it generates at its peak continue to benefit your body. After two days of Ketosis, it will be obvious that you have done good for your health.

After 48 hours of Ketosis, you get a great influx of growth hormones. From the name alone, you might not think growth hormones would be something you want more of, but they actually are. The more growth hormones you have, the easier time your body has keeping fat tissues from accumulating.

You might think that two days gives you plenty of Ketosis and autophagy. You may feel that you get plenty of benefits from going through Ketosis for just this long.

But you need to remember that Keto requires you to stick with it. You will simply gain the weight back again if you don't follow the Ketogenic lifestyle any longer.

Besides, one of the best health benefits happens at 54 hours. When you are in Ketosis for 54 hours, you start to get to an insulin level that is still safe and healthy, but also very low. With low insulin, the enzyme mTOR is suppressed.

In order to keep your autophagy as engaged as possible, you always want to keep mTOR down. Insulin is connected to mTOR, and a low activation of mTOR leads to more autophagy.

Your insulin will be at its lowest (therefore keeping autophagy in an advanced stage) when mTOR is low. You keep your insulin low by not putting outside food sources into your body.

In other words, 54 hours into Ketosis, your metabolism is going to be more efficient than ever.

To reset your metabolism, you will want to pair your Ketogenic diet with a lifestyle that increases autophagy.

You already know how Keto works, but if you want to increase your autophagy, you will want to decrease the window of time during which you eat every day.

This means following the Keto diet, eating your Ketogenic meals at the same time each day, and not eating any snacks outside of these windows of time. If you do that, you will push your metabolism to be more efficient than it has ever been.

Chapter 7: Keto FAQs

This chapter will answer common questions about Keto that aren't covered in the rest of the book. The answers will help you feel more confident about what you are getting into before you take the plunge.

How long will it take for my system to go into Ketosis after I start my new diet?

It depends. Some people can tell they are in a state of Ketosis after just 3 or 4 days because of their physical changes. For others, it can take up to 2 weeks. Either way, you will certainly notice a difference in at least a couple of weeks.

Should I track my carb intake while I am in Keto?

Of course, you should keep track of your carbs, because when it comes down to it, your carb intake is what Keto is all about.

You would be surprised how many carbs you eat every day without even realizing it. It is hard to notice this in the hustle and bustle of everyday life—the only way you will start to notice is by logging your carb intake in your journal. If you aren't marking it down, you just aren't going to notice it as much.

This goes for life in general. People don't pay attention to things like their carb consumption if they don't write it down. They eat snacks all throughout the day that are high in carbs, but since it is just a snack here and there, they don't realize how much these add up in their carb consumption.

If you don't want to write in a journal, there are plenty of apps out there that can do the same thing. You may find this to be more convenient.

However, I have a piece of advice regarding using apps with Keto. Don't fall into the trap of thinking you are doing Keto because you are using an app.

When we use a Keto app, it makes us feel like we are doing everything right. It doesn't matter if we aren't meeting our weight loss goals or following the actual Ketogenic guidelines. Simply having the app on our phone makes it feel like we are living the Keto lifestyle.

That's one of the reasons why I would recommend you writing a Keto journal instead of using an app. Plus, it feels more personal and tactile to write down words with ink on paper than it does to interact with a phone app. That said, whatever helps you achieve your Keto goals is fine.

Do I need to track my calories?

A lot of women figure they don't need to track calories while on Keto. The hard truth is that with Keto, just like with any diet, calories are very important. You still have to track with calories when you are on Keto. You can do this on your app or in your Keto journal.

An exciting part of counting calories is that you can also subtract them from your Keto journal or app when you do exercise. I include a chapter about exercises for women to do while they are on Keto for a reason: exercise is a vital part of a healthy lifestyle.

You should never look at Keto as a cure-all for your health. Keto is one of many things you should be doing to watch your health. The key things in your general health will always be diet, exercise, and mental health.

Mental health is something that requires its own book to dive into, but I focus on the Keto diet in the rest of the chapters and exercise in the last. The exercises provided to you in Chapter 10 were chosen because they are simple to follow, while still giving your body the workout it needs to make the most out of your new Ketogenic lifestyle.

As much as I want to stress the significance of calories in and calories out, I also don't want to give the false impression that it is always simple. After all, bodies are different from person to person. What works for one individual does not always work for the next.

There are simply too many different factors to consider. Genetics obviously play a large role in the bodies we have. They help determine our metabolisms, allergies, and endocrine disorders, all of which can influence body shape and size.

It doesn't mean you should give in to whatever body you are naturally given. Anyone can achieve the body and health goals they want if they are willing to put in the extra time and work.

Don't eat too many calories in the first place. Offset your extra calories by burning them with exercise. Don't let exercise become an excuse for you to eat non-Ketogenic snack foods, either.

It may be a hard thing to commit to, but you will not be able to enter Ketosis without completely eliminating these snack foods from your diet. All you can really do is say "No" to these snack foods.

At the same time, don't overthink calories when you are doing Keto. Getting most of your calories from healthy fats and proteins will consistently get you the calories you need.

If you exercise a lot, you will notice that you have to eat more than you used to. If you don't, you will run into a calorie deficit and run out of energy.

Now, let's move on to the next common concern of new Keto practitioners.

Won't the fats I eat in Keto make me gain weight?

The reasoning behind this question is logical. We get told our entire lives that people who put on too much weight are eating too much fat. We are told not to eat too many fats, so we don't gain weight.

But as you've learned from this book, that simply isn't the case. People gain weight because they eat too many calories from a wide variety of sources—carbs, saturated fats, and excessive protein—and then don't burn those calories off with exercise.

It is hard to get away from that misconception, because we are told our whole lives that fat is the problem. To get out of this misconception, you need to remember that fat itself is not the problem. Nutritionists will tell you that fat is not the problem. The problem is eating too many calories from these three sources, and then not exercising.

If you get healthy, unsaturated fats, few carbs, and just enough protein, you will have a much better outlook for your weight and for your health.

Can you get too much fat on Keto?

Yes, there is such a thing as eating too much fat on Keto. But it is not the fat itself that is the problem. It is the calories we put into our bodies without burning them for energy.

Another way to look at this is through the lens of carbs. People say that eating too many fats is the problem. It is called fat, after all. But don't forget this is a different kind of fat than the body fat that builds up, making you gain weight and appear larger.

In fact, fats are not usually the nutrients that add up to the caloric surplus that makes us gain weight. Usually, it is carbs.

The answer to the question is technically yes, but the truth is, avoiding eating too many carbs will help you more than avoiding fats.

How much weight will I lose if I do the Keto diet?

I wish there were a simple answer on this one, but the most I can do is provide you a way to find out as best as you can.

Don't get sidetracked by focusing so much on your goal weight. If you focus all your attention on where you want to be and not what you are doing today, you won't be able to make the necessary changes.

You already know what to do from reading along—the hard part is putting it into action. We all know that we will lose more weight if we exercise more. We all know we will lose weight if we eat fewer calories. These things are not hard to understand; they are just hard to follow through on.

Because of the power of Ketosis itself, I can tell you that you can expect to lose a few pounds—at the least—in as little as a few days into Keto. You will continue to see these results if you stick with the program.

Chapter 8: Doing Keto as a Woman Over 50

Many women want to lose weight, but women over the age of 50 are particularly interested in losing weight, boosting their immune system, and having more energy.

If you fit into this group, this chapter will address the particular hurdles you may face when doing the Keto diet. For one thing, women in this age range experience slowing metabolisms, making it harder to drop pounds than ever before.

I will cover the tweaks you can make to your Keto diet and lifestyle to accommodate these particular hurdles. I will address any concerns you may have and give you solutions to counteract them.

Women go through menopause sometime between the ages of 45 and 55, and it can be a particularly difficult time. They notice they are putting on weight, and they experience all kinds of unpleasant symptoms such as difficulty sleeping and hot flashes.

But many of these symptoms are temporary. The one that bothers women the most is the one that lasts: weight gain. Women over 50 want to know how they can stave off weight gain and lose the extra pounds they started to put on after menopause.

First of all, I highly recommend intermittent fasting for women in this age group. Intermittent fasting is often paired with Keto for the best possible results in autophagy. Autophagy can be improved through Keto alone, but you don't truly unlock the potential advanced autophagy in your body until you fast between your Ketogenic meals.

The reason I urge you to do intermittent fasting with Keto is because it will help you more with the effects of aging than Keto alone. The autophagy that results from fasting doesn't only help you get better skin, lose weight, and detox your cells—although all these things are worth trying to achieve on their own.

The long-term, anti-aging benefits of intermittent fasting are more important but often ignored. The autophagy that comes from intermittent fasting will help you lower your inflammation, boost your metabolism, enhance your immune system, and more. These are all benefits of autophagy that are backed by scientific research.

Studies show time and time again that fasting works to help women lose weight and improve their health. As a woman over 50, you should consider doing Keto together with fasting.

Scientists are not in agreement about whether menopause itself affects weight. Some say that when women gain weight at this stage in life, it is because of aging alone. They do not believe the hormonal changes from menopause are the reason for the weight gain.

But there is no denying that the lowered estrogen from menopause has some impact on the distribution of fat on the body of a woman over 50. You may have noticed this yourself in your own body: the change in hormones tends to make a woman's fat go from her hips to her waist.

That isn't all, either. Women who go through menopause also report that they have less energy and have a harder time burning fat. It is no wonder women over 50 want to know how to lose weight. It is such a harder feat at this stage in life.

But don't be misled to believe the change in metabolism is all that is going on here. After all, a doctor studying women over 50 found that women's bodies only metabolized 50 calories fewer calories every day. While this is not a negligible figure, it can hardly be blamed for all of the weight gain that is experienced by women at this age.

You are sure to have experienced some of the other factors that play into weight gain for women at this age. Women over 50 report having more cravings, doing less exercise, and losing more muscle.

As you might guess, many of these factors are related. When you aren't exercising as much, you won't retain as much muscle. If you have more cravings for foods you shouldn't eat, you are more likely to eat those foods and gain weight as a result.

Top it all off with the less efficient metabolisms of women over 50, and it is easy to understand why they have a hard time losing weight. Even if menopause itself isn't the reason women experience this, it all adds up to make weight loss seem impossible, if you don't know anything about Keto or fasting.

Take everything you hear them say about weight gain for women over 50 with a grain of salt. All of us know that it is a reality for women who fall into this age range, but no one knows exactly what the reason for it is. But we do know that Keto and fasting both show fantastic results for these women, so that is the information we should really be paying attention to.

Women in this age range can still go wrong when they try Keto and autophagy, so I have some pieces of advice to give you if you count yourself among this group.

The first piece of advice is to make sure you eat enough protein every day. You might be worried about eating too much protein because you are watching calories, and this is a reasonable thing to do. But when you are on Keto, you need protein as a source of energy.

It is always about balance. On the one hand, you need to make up for the energy you won't be getting from carbs. On the other hand, you have to be careful not to eat too many calories.

As usual, follow along with what your body is telling you. If your body tells you that you still need more energy, wait a bit. You can eat more if some time passes and you still feel hungry.

That probably means you need the food for energy. But you have to give yourself this waiting period because otherwise, your mind might be trying to trick you into just eating something you are craving when you are not genuinely hungry.

There is a mental component to this change in diet, too. The problem at the center of women not being able to change their diet is not being used to the real feeling of being full.

By the "real" feeling of being full, I am referring to how people feel when they have eaten enough—not too much.

These days, people eat so many carbs that their idea of fullness is the uncomfortable feeling they have when they eat too many carbs. But you can't lose weight if you see fullness this way. You will consistently overstuff yourself, believing you are making yourself full when you are actually gorging yourself.

To remind yourself what fullness actually feels like, get used to eating without overstuffing yourself. Get used to not feeling uncomfortable after eating. It can feel strangely comforting to be overstuffed with carbs, but that is not a feeling we can let ourselves get used to. If we do, we will never be happy with the simple feeling of fullness.

As I keep emphasizing, we can't villainize fat anymore. The real problem is eating too many calories, most of which tend to come from carbs, not fats. However, women over 50, in particular, need to be careful not to eat too many fats when they follow Keto.

Keto isn't a valid excuse for simply eating a ton of fat. You still need to show some constraint as you do in every diet.

Understanding how to balance your fat consumption will take understanding how fat fits into Keto. With Keto, you want to be what we call fat-adapted.

You already know what this means; it is just another way of saying what happens in Ketosis. Being fat-adapted means, you are burning fat for energy with Ketones instead of burning glucose with carbs.

I tell you this term because you should eat a lot of healthy fats until you go through significant Ketosis—until you are fat-adapted. Once that happens, you should start being more careful with how much fat you are consuming.

One of the sources women over 50 will get fat from is drinks. Even the drinks you make at home like coffee with milk can be a lot higher in fat than you think. It should go without saying that the specialty coffee you get topped with whipped cream is high in fat.

Women over 50 know they have their own hurdles to overcome when they chase the goals of weight loss and improved overall health with Keto. But they can do all they can possibly do by following along with the advice in this chapter.

Chapter 9:
How to Have More Energy

Women who start the Keto diet notice a newfound surge of energy. The influx of Ketones causes their body to burn fat as a new source of energy, giving them more energy than they ever thought they had. At the same time, women who do Keto sometimes have to grapple with a phenomenon known as the Keto flu. Women who go through the Keto flu feel like they have no energy.

The Keto flu happens because women's bodies are readjusting to the new source of energy—they doesn't always adjust quickly, leading to the Keto flu. However, in time you will definitely feel the increase of energy, even if you experience the Keto flu at first.

This chapter will tell you how to avoid the Keto flu and how to handle it if you go through it. It also tells you how to optimize your surge of energy while on Keto.

First, we need to fully address the controversial issue of the Keto flu.

Of all the negative aspects of Keto, the Keto flu is easily the most well-known. The Keto flu is a series of symptoms that show up a few days into starting the Keto diet.

The symptoms include irritation, tiredness, trouble thinking, constipation, and migraines. Since Keto itself is still relatively new, the Keto flu is not very well studied or understood. Everything we know about it is from the personal experience of women who have tried the Ketogenic diet.

We also can't attribute all the symptoms to Keto with 100% accuracy, making it particularly hard to study. After all, women who do Keto may be cutting out processed food from their diet for the first time. It could be that the more natural foods are causing these symptoms—not Ketosis.

Ketosis might be the goal of Keto, but achieving it requires you to make drastic lifestyle changes. These drastic lifestyle changes could lead to these symptoms on their own.

Maybe a woman experiences the symptoms of Keto flu because they went through the most advanced autophagy she ever has. It could be the lowered carb intake by itself and not the influx of Ketones that results from it. The Keto flu doesn't even happen to everyone—it may not happen to you at all.

The worst consequence of the Keto flu is that women get discouraged and give up on the Ketogenic diet altogether. It is extremely unfortunate, given how much Keto could have done for their weight loss and health. But when the first thing you experience with a diet is fatigue and sickness, it isn't surprising that you might not want to do it anymore.

Whatever you do, steer clear of anything labeled "Keto" that you find in the store, whether it is a supplement or a food. With the popularity Keto has been gaining, corporations have been rushing to profit off of it with products that don't help achieve Ketosis at all. People buy them simply because they say Keto on them.

We can feel tempted to get these products when we know about the Keto flu. We want to eliminate any feeling of discomfort that might accompany a change of diet. But the fact is, that discomfort is a reality of dieting that you will have to accept.

You will know the difference between mere discomfort and actual sickness. Don't let yourself believe you are sick to get out of doing Keto—you know in the back of your mind that you are fine. Even when you are eating foods that are better for you, it can be hard to physically adjust to a new diet. The Keto flu is an adjustment to the new group of chemicals appearing in your body.

Any trace of the Keto flu should only last a couple days, at most. If it lasts any longer, you could actually be sick. Reach out to a doctor if this happens.

There are measures you can take to prevent Keto flu and to cope with it better when you have it.

You should do two important things to deal with Keto flu: (1) hydrate plenty with lots of water and (2) eat as many Keto-friendly vegetables as you can. Everyone knows how important water is in your body, and eating vegetables is to help your system adjust by giving it the nutrients it needs.

The next and last piece of advice I have on the Keto flu is more on the mental side of things. You might feel ready to give up on Keto completely after experiencing the Keto flu, but I urge you not to give in to this feeling.

It will be very tempting to simply go back to what you did before you heard of Keto: allowing your body to be filled with tons of carbs every day that just make you gain weight and become less healthy.

The best way to avoid this temptation is to know what you want out of Keto from the beginning.

Your Keto journal is not only a tool to mark down your exercise and diet habits. You should also write out your short-term and long-term goals as well. You can get what you are looking for out of Keto, even if it isn't easy right away. You just have to be willing to stick with it through the most challenging days.

Carbs are the main events of the typical America's diet. Even when the main part of your meal is not carb-heavy, there's usually something carb-heavy on the side. For example, a low-carb meat might have mashed potatoes as the side, which are carb-heavy. One of the biggest problems with carbs is how deleterious they are to our energy levels.

When you consume a lot of carbohydrates, the starches are turned into glucose during digestion. You get a burst of energy from this glucose when you consume carbs. At that point, it doesn't seem like a high-carb diet gives you any trouble with your energy levels. But the issue is, when your system burns carbs for fuel, it has to use insulin transport the energy to your cells, which are what actually need the energy.

The problem for many women is they develop insulin resistance from their high-carb diets, even when they don't become diabetic. Because of this, they will get a short surge of energy after eating their high carb meals, and then immediately lose all of that energy.

It turns into a vicious cycle. You start to think that the short burst of energy is what energy has to be. You seek out more carbs for energy to get these short bursts instead of seeking out the longer, more sustained energy that is possible with the Ketogenic diet.

When we start to adapt Keto into our daily routine, we realize we don't need to constantly eat high-carb snacks to have energy. We realize it is far more sustainable to eat low-carb foods for energy and spread this energy out through the day.

The way many people live in America today, they think it is normal to get their energy from carbs. But now you know this is simply untrue. It isn't the carbs themselves that are providing us with energy, but the sugar our bodies make from the carbs.

But we end up needing more and more of these carbs repeatedly, like a drug. You may know from experience how this cycle of carb dependence can easily lead to eating too much.

Did you know that most Americans get over half of their calories from carbs? From the popular perception, you would think that most Americans would get their calories from fat. But it is actually carbs that make up most of the clarities of the average American.

Specifically, most Americans get over 220 grams of carbohydrates into their systems every day. Take a moment to let that soak in.

Thankfully, you don't have to continue being dependent on carbs any longer. You know you can make your body fat-adapted, so it is used to burning fat for energy instead of carbs, making you feel full of energy instead of sluggish and tired the way carbs do.

The best part is, you won't constantly crave more food to get energy. Carbs count on you to constantly crave more of them when you rely on them for energy. But fat as energy is much more sustainable, so you can just eat a good meal or two a day that is high in unsaturated fats and protein, and low in carbs. It will hold you over for the rest of the day. You won't feel hungry or tired like you would if you depended on carbs for fuel.

Once you get over the initial Keto flu—if you're one of the few people who experience that at all—you will be able to enjoy the great increase in your energy levels in about 4 days to a week.

With carbs as your energy source, you only feel energetic when you are eating carbs. Ketosis allows you to feel energized as long as you have been eating well. Every day, eat two or more meals that follow the Keto guidelines; you will notice you have enough energy to do anything you put your mind to.

To address the issue of hormones in Keto again, it is worth noting that you may want to eat a little more protein and healthy fats during the third and fourth weeks of your cycle. This is the period where your cravings are at their worst, so you will be most tempted to consume carbs for energy then.

Chapter 10:
Best Exercises to Lose Weight

Dieticians and physical health professionals recommend certain exercise practices for women going through Keto. This chapter puts all of these recommended exercises in one place so you won't have to look anywhere else.

To start out, know that you shouldn't do any exercises that are too high in intensity. You don't want to strain your system while it is adjusting to its new source of energy—this will only harm you in the long run. You may want to lose as much weight as quickly as possible, but exercising constantly and at too high levels of intensity is not good for your body either.

Exercise is the best method of increasing the quality and length of your life at the same time. Even if you weren't trying to lose, exercise would be a good thing to pick up. After all, the older you get, the harder it gets for your body to do all the ordinary things that you used to take for granted. Exercise helps you make the most of the body you have.

Every study ever done about exercise shows that it helps women stay healthy. It can help maintain the health of all your organs, including your skin, heart, and lungs.

There is one particular kind of exercise that is most important for women over 50. This is strength training.

Strength training helps women maintain muscle tone, as you would expect, but that isn't all it does. Strength training shines the most in how it can directly trigger autophagy. Overall, strength training exercises are one of the best things you can do for your body.

Exercise is very hard to get people to do at any age, but it is especially important for people over 50 to get into strength training. By this point in life, it isn't about getting abs or toned arms. It is about keeping your muscles engaged so you can continue to use them for practical purposes.

The statistics on muscle loss paint a clear picture. One study demonstrated that adults between 30 and 80 lose up to forty percent of their strength if they are sedentary.

Keeping your existing muscle mass doesn't mean you have to turn into some sort of superhero. It just means you can do normal things around the house, do your own shopping, take care of your lawn, and get up when you fall.

Your muscle mass isn't all that matters here. Keeping up with strength training also maintains the density of your bones. Women over 50 need to be particularly cognizant of their bone density. When you have more fragile bones, you are at a much higher risk of injury when you fall down. When we are young, our bones are sturdy and elastic. We could repeatedly fall without any issues. But the older we get, the riskier it is to fall, because you may be at serious risk of injury.

Strength training will also help you burn fat. It won't do it as quickly as cardiovascular training, such as running on a treadmill, but it is better for you in other ways besides just losing weight.

I don't want to discount the health benefits associated with losing weight itself, either. Being at a healthy weight puts you at a much lower risk for any age-related disease, so having a lower body weight is the best thing you can have when you are older.

We shouldn't ignore the psychological benefits of strength training. Studies show that older adults who exercise regularly have higher self-confidence and lower rates of depression.

All it takes is about half an hour of strength training every day, and you will be able to enjoy all these benefits. Now that you have a strong grasp on all the benefits, let's get started.

Several workouts include single-leg moves or stability ball moves. These particular workouts were included to help improve balance and coordination. These two things both become harder to maintain with age, so they are important to watch for.

The only equipment you need for these exercises are hand weights of a weight that is not too heavy and a stability ball. You can get any of these supplies for very cheap at your local supermarket.

You don't necessarily need to do the stability ball exercises with the ball, however. It will help you improve balance if you use the ball, but you can also do the exercises on the floor.

Do 8-12 repetitions for every work out and give yourself a 30-60 second break in between reps. Take your time with each of them, and be sure to get in deep breaths throughout all of them. Don't take it too seriously: allow yourself to enjoy it and take it at your own pace. Do not stress about these workouts.

If you have a group, you can work out with, reach out to them. You can join a class if you don't know anyone who might be interested in working out together.

Forearm Plan

Engage your core and raise your body up off the floor, keeping your forearms on the floor and your body in a straight line from head to feet. Keep your abdominals engaged and try not to let your hips rise or drop. Instead of 8-12 reps, hold for 30 seconds. If it hurts your low back or becomes too difficult, place your knees down on the ground.

Targets: shoulders, core

Modified Push-Up

Begin in a kneeling position on a mat with hands below shoulders and knees behind hips so back is angled and long.

Tuck toes under, tighten abdominals, and bend elbows to lower chest toward the floor. Keep your gaze in front of your fingertips, so neck stays long.

Press chest back up to starting position.

Targets: shoulders, arm, core

Basic Squat

Stand tall with your feet hip-distance apart. Your hips, knees, and toes should all be facing forward. (Hold dumbbells in hands to make it harder).

Bend your knees and extend your buttocks backward as if you are going to sit back into a chair. Make sure that you keep your knees behind your toes and your weight in your heels. Rise back up and repeat.

Targets: glutes, quads, hamstrings

Stability Ball Chest Fly

Hold a pair of dumbbells close to your chest and place your shoulder blades, and head on top of the ball with the rest of your body in a tabletop position. Feet should be hip-distance apart.

Raise dumbbells together straight above the chest, palms facing in.

Slowly lower arms out to the side with a slight bend in your elbow, until elbows are about chest level.

Squeeze chest and bring hands back together at the top.

Targets: chest, glutes, back, core

Stability Ball Tricep Kick Back

Holding dumbbells, place your chest on the ball with arms draped alongside the ball and legs extended out to the floor behind you. Keep head in line with your spine. (If you don't have a ball, lay belly-side down on a bench or stand with feet staggered from to back and body hinged forward).

Pull your elbow up to a 90-degree angle for start position.

Press dumbbells back to lengthen arms, squeezing triceps.

Release dumbbells back down to start position.

Targets: triceps, core

Shoulder Overhead Press

Start with feet hip-distance apart. Bring elbows out to the side, creating a goal post position with arms, dumbbells are at the side of the head, and abdominals are tight.

Press dumbbells slowly up until arms are straight. Slowly return to starting position with control. If desired, you can also perform this exercise seated in a chair or on a stability ball with feet wide.

Targets: shoulders, biceps, back

Stability Ball Overhead Pull

Hold a pair of dumbbells close to your chest and place your shoulder blades, and head on top of the ball with the rest of your body in a tabletop position. Feet should be hip-distance apart.

Raise dumbbells together straight above the chest, palms facing in.

Slowly lower arms behind the back of your head, keeping only a slight bend in your elbows.

Squeeze your lats as you pull arms back to start position above the chest.

Targets: back, core

Stability Ball Side Leg Lift

Begin kneeling with the ball to your right side.

Let your right side lean slightly on the ball and hug your right arm around the ball.

Extend left leg long to the side. The right leg should remain bent on the floor.

Slowly lift and lower left leg 8-12 times, then switch sides.

Targets: legs, core

Single-Leg Hamstring Bridge

Lie on back with bent knees hip-distance apart, and feet flat on meat

Squeeze glutes and lift hips off the mat into a bridge. Lower and lift the hips for 8-12 reps then repeat on the other side.

Targets: hamstrings, glutes, quads

Bird Dog

Kneel on the mat on all fours.

Reach one arm long, draw in the abdominals, and extend the opposite leg long behind you.

Repeat 8-12 times then switch sides.

Conclusion

Thank you for making it through to the end of *Keto Diet for Women over 50*, let's hope it was informative and able to provide you with all of the tools you need to achieve your goals whatever they may be.

You've come a long way to get to this page. Now, you know how to make a plan for changing your eating habits; you know how your lifestyle changes will affect you differently as a woman over 50.

You read all our advice on avoiding the common mistakes women make when they are first starting out with the Ketogenic diet. We even went over special exercises that women say help them in their health goals.

Now, your job is to take it from theory to practice. You know all you need to know—only you can make the necessary changes for yourself.

I suspect that the section you will get the most use out of is the 30-day meal plan for Keto. Don't feel like you can't stray away from these recipes, however. There are, in fact, other meals outside of this list that still accord to the requirements of the Keto diet. You can simply use the recipes on this list to come up with meals of your own, and make modifications as you see fit.

The biggest problem that women have after getting invested in Keto is continuing to follow through with their plans. They get inspired to get into it and even do everything right for weeks or even months.

But then something inevitably happens in their life that makes Keto a lower priority. The key to prevent this from happening to you is keeping a Keto journal.

In your Keto journal, you will keep yourself accountable for your diet and exercise goals. All of them go together to get the results you are looking for: the foods you eat every day and the amount of time you spend in the gym are both things you should write down in your Keto journal.

Many women will be very hesitant to do this. Mainly, they are concerned they will start the journal only to end up leaving it behind. But the first few weeks is when the Keto journal matters the most.

You should try to keep up with it as long as you can, but even if you end up leaving it behind later, the Keto journal will be a great help to commit yourself to Keto. After all, you have your commitments to the lifestyle written on paper.

In a similar way, the exercises I give you in the last chapter will help you feel committed to Keto. This is because, as with the Keto journal, these exercises get your body engaged in this new lifestyle. With the journal, you get your hands involved in Keto as they write out your progress. With the exercises, the rest of your body gets involved. It is a perfect way to demonstrate to yourself that you are really in this for the long haul.

My final note to you is to be forgiving of yourself. No one—not a single soul—starts the Keto lifestyle and stick with it without making any mistakes. It is no different from any other change that people make to their lives, in this sense.

People who quit smoking for months often find themselves cheating and smoking a cigarette, and they end up picking up cigarettes more and more after that, thinking they have already messed up irredeemably.

This is because we are so used to sticking with our new routine that breaking away from it with our old habits makes it feel like we are getting back to our old selves.

Don't let yourself fall into this trap. Accept right now that you will make a mistake at some point. You will eat a non-Keto food; you won't go to the gym on a day you said you would; you won't follow the fasting routine you have set for yourself.

Whatever the goals you set for yourself, you can't be a complete perfectionist about them. Be open to your lifestyle change while also being open to slipping ever now and again.

Finally, if you found this book useful in any way, a review on Amazon is always appreciated!

Meal Prep for Beginners

A Complete Meal Prep Cookbook: Your Essential Guide to Losing Weight With Many Easy Recipes, a 30-Day meal plan for weight loss, and Ideas for Healthy Meals to Prep and Go!

Jason Watchers

Introduction

Congratulations on purchasing *Meal Prep for Beginners: A Complete Meal Prep Cookbook – Your Essential Guide To Losing Weight and Saving Time – Many Quick and Easy Recipes, 30 Day Meal Plan to Weight Loss, And Healthy Meals To Prep and Go!* and thank you for doing so.

The following chapters will discuss how you can learn the basics of meal prep and then move on to prepping your meals for the entire month with the goal of losing weight. When it comes to the fitness world, meal prepping is the to-go solution for so many people because it not only makes your life easier by saving time, but it also helps in portion control. When it comes to losing weight fast, it is meal prep that is going to go a long way in helping you to achieve your goals.

If you are just a beginner, you need not worry as meal prepping is not something difficult. Rather, meeting your body's dietary needs has never been easier, and all you need is a little bit of planning. Meal prepping will help you in maintaining your diet successfully and at the same time, you can stay stress-free because all the meals for the week have already been prepared. When a process is time-consuming, that is when it is easier for you to give up on your diet but the idea behind meal prepping is to make things much less complex.

There are plenty of books on this subject on the market, thanks again for choosing this one! Every effort was made to ensure it is full of as much useful information as possible; please enjoy!

Chapter 1: What is Prepping?

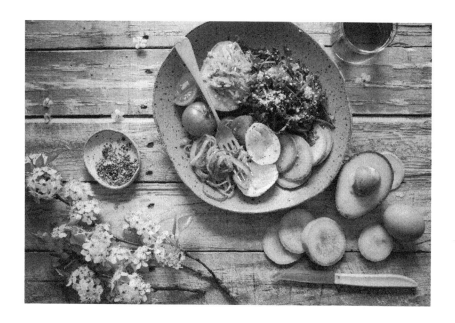

As you might have understood from the name itself, meal prepping is all about preparing your meals for the next few days or for the week ahead of time so that you don't have to worry about it during the week. The idea of meal prepping is gaining even more momentum in today's world, where everyone is so busy in their lives. Controlling the portion size is one of the biggest struggles faced by every person who has just started limiting his/her calories in a day. But with meal prepping, you can get help with that too.

Since you already have your meal prepared so it will become easier to fight the urge or ordering takeout after a long day at work. You can simply take out one of the meal prep containers from the refrigerator and put it in the microwave. Your dinner is ready, and do you know what the best part about this is? You are getting healthy, homemade food instead of all the junk you would have gulped down otherwise. In case of meal prepping, you actually have to decide your meals from way before and this is also one of the reasons why people end up eating healthy because they are consciously making healthier choices for the week ahead.

Most people have this wrong notion about meal prepping whereby they think that they have to spend their entire Sunday cooking just so they can eat healthy throughout the week. But that is where you are wrong. Meal prepping is all about making life easier, and it definitely does not involve taking away your one holiday from you. You don't necessarily have to prepare the entire week's meal in a day. You can prep your meals twice a week – once on a Sunday and once on a Thursday or Wednesday and in this way, you will be able to divide the work between these two days in a week. So, it is basically in your hands as to how you want to divide your work.

One of the best aspects of meal prepping is the make-ahead breakfasts because they tend to make your morning routine streamlined, and you literally have all the time you need to get ready. You can also try batch-cooked meals especially if you are someone who returns late or exhausted on most days and you don't have the energy to make something for yourself. So, at the end of the day, it depends on your circumstances and which method appeals to your situation the best.

Now, you might be wondering whether you can meal prep every type of food or not. Well, since meal prep involved storing the food in a refrigerator in air-tight containers and then reheating before eating, some of the items that are well-suited for meal prep are soups, roasted vegetables, cooked meat, nuts and stiff, sauces, and even raw veggies. But, on the other hand, if you are meal prepping crunchy food, after a certain point of time, no matter how well you store them, they are going to get soggy.

Chapter 2:
10 Reasons Why
You Should Meal Prep

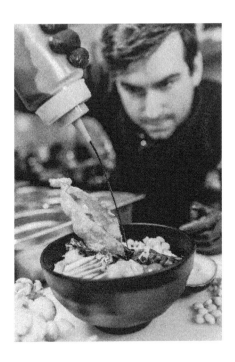

If you are not aware of all the reasons as to why meal prepping is a viable option for anyone, then this chapter should walk you through. Everyone had faced situations in their life when they came home tired and exhausted, and instead of making something at home ended up ordering takeout. But is that healthy? No. So, meal prepping provides you an easier way out of the cycle of takeouts and quick fixes. Here are ten reasons why you should incorporate meal prepping in your weekly routine.

Better Control on Portions

If you want a healthy and balanced meal, controlling your portions is of utmost significance. And what if I tell you that the solution to your problem is right in front of you? You don't believe me, right? Well, it is none other than meal prepping. Most people would tell you to use kitchen scales or measuring cups, but meal prepping involves using storage containers that are compartmentalized. And since you are planning your meals beforehand, you know how many calories you include in a day.

Save Money

Now, you might be wondering how exactly you are saving money when you have to buy things for making the food. Well, when you are going out to eat somewhere, you will spend at least $8-$10 in the fast-food counters, and the same goes for when you are ordering the food. But for that same amount of money, you can make almost half a week of meals. Also, meal prepping involves sticking to two to three types of meals in a week which means that you do not need a whole lot of varied ingredients and so you won't be wasting any money. You will not be using the dishwasher as frequently as you used to before since you are prepping the meals on one or two days for the entire week. So, you will be saving on your energy bill too.

Improve Your Skills in Cooking

With meal prepping, you will get to learn a whole range of recipes. You don't have to try them all out at once. Start with something simple, and if you are just a beginner, stick to a few recipes and then you can work your way up from there. But at the end of the day, you will learn new recipes. For those who did not know much about cooking, the desire to eat healthily will also give you the chance to brush up on your cooking skills and what better way than meal prep.

Eliminate Hidden Calories

Hidden calories are the reason why people end up sabotaging their diets, even when everything seems to be going well. The most common reason for hidden calories is mindless eating. There are times when people consume calories without even knowing that they are doing so. This happens especially when people grab drinks to satiate their cravings or hunger. A beverage can easily spike up your net calorie intake way more than solid food. Also, when people are always on the go, they simply grab something from a nearby fast-food counter or take an energy bar along with them. What you don't realize is that fast-food might contain a lot of trans fat or simply unwanted calories because of the extra cheese toppings. Or, that energy bar you are having might contain fructose syrup which is unhealthy. That is why meal prepping can help you as you can prep some snacks that can be easily carried in your bag in a small container and will be your savior when you are hungry.

Save Time

Meal prepping makes life incredibly easy, and you have to plan your days based on when you want to go to the supermarket to buy the ingredients and when you want to prep the meals. So, everything in your calendar is sorted out. You will also get apps that keep the ingredients list assorted for you. Now, when you complete everything as planned, you will have all the meals for the coming week prepared in your refrigerator and the time you previously used in preparing meals every day will be left for you to do whatever you want.

Better Results from Workouts

Workouts alone will not yield you the desired results if you do not control what you eat. Meal prepping will assist you with that. This will make those strenuous gym sessions worth all the sweat. If you have planned on achieving your desired results within a particular span of time, then meal prepping will help you reach your goals faster. You won't be snacking when you are not supposed to, and you won't be going past your set calorie limits for the day. In short, your exercise will visibly show the results you so wanted.

Come Home to a Nice Meal

Everyone loves to come back after a long day at work to a sumptuous homemade meal but not everyone can make it happen especially because of all the stress and how tired they are by the time they reach home. Thus, you won't end up ordering any junk food from outside or worse – go to sleep on an empty stomach. With meal prepping, you will have your favorite food waiting for you in the refrigerator and all you have to do is pop it into the refrigerator, reheat and enjoy!

Variety In Your Meals

This is also one of the biggest reasons why you should meal prep. It helps in bringing variety to your food, which means that you are not only keeping your taste buds pleased but you are also getting a properly balanced diet. Since you are planning your meals beforehand in case of meal prep, you get to make a choice from among the several food categories available to you. There is no one stopping you from mixing it up in a new way every week. You can get creative with your food as much as you want. Meal prepping might mean getting more organized but it does not make food monotonous. In fact, it is quite the opposite!

Increase Your Willpower

Once you make meal prepping a habit, it will become easier, and gradually, you will also notice that you do not crave sugary foods or junk foods like you used to before. Healthy eating is all about setting a routine and then sticking to it. With time, even when someone asks you to eat something that you know is unhealthy, you will know how to say 'no.' And, when others see your commitment to a healthier lifestyle, it will encourage them to do the same as well. Thus, you become an inspiration for others which further strengthens your willpower.

No More Food Wastage

Since you are making a list of all the meals you are going to prepare and the ingredients you need to for them, you do not end up wasting any food. There have been times in everyone's life when they had to throw away something before even tasting it just because they didn't have the time to eat. So, meal prepping prevents all of that as it involved preparing selective meals for specific times and so, nothing goes to waste and you end up saving money that way too.

Chapter 3:
Tips and Tricks to Make Meal Prepping Easier

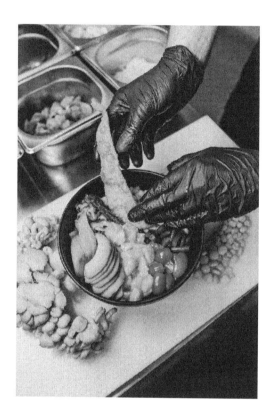

When it comes to maintaining your personal health and making a conscious choice about heating healthy, meal prepping is the best option. So, if you want to have a successful meal prepping strategy at hand, here are some tips and tricks that you should follow.

Don't Stuff Too Many Things At a Time

If you are someone who took a long hiatus from meal prepping but now are getting back to it or is you are starting it for the first time, there will be times when you might feel overwhelmed with the process. It can be a daunting thing, but think of it like any other positive habit you want to inculcate in your routine. Any big change in a person's life always starts with you taking a small step towards it. This helps in building the confidence one step at a time. When you start small, you can also make the habit sustainable. You should not be making things so big that you are not able to sustain it on an everyday basis.

So, in the case of meal prepping, start by preparing some snacks or simple breakfasts for the upcoming week or for the next two to three days. Then, after a few weeks have passed, you will know which meal combination works best for you or which strategies suit your needs. Also, you can tweak your plans accordingly based on whether you want more variety or stick to more basic meals.

Be Organized

If you want your meal plan to be successful, then one of the first things that you need to ensure is that you are well-organized. Meal prep will seem like a breeze when everything is in place starting from your refrigerator to your pantry and even your kitchen. One of the first things that you can do is check your fridge and toss out anything that you find hasn't been touched or used in months or has already expired. You should also take all the unhealthy food items and either distribute them among your friends who would take it or simply keep them in some other place away from your eyes. Once you have simplified your fridge, you will have a clear idea of what exactly you need.

Another key idea to help in improving your organizational skills is to group your ingredients when you are planning the meals. For example, there will be some ingredients that are required by multiple recipes. So, you need to keep them side by side. Also, prefer clear containers over solid containers because of one simple reason – you can easily see what is inside and thus make decisions faster. You don't always have to open the containers to see what's inside them. Sometimes, mason jars can work pretty well in certain scenarios. Also, it is a good idea to put on a label on your containers where you will write down the date on which you have prepared the food so that you can keep track of the leftovers and till when you can consume it safely.

Keep Each Food Group in Mind

This is another very important step that people often forget. Whether you are meal prepping for just the next few days or the entire month, your plan should have every food group, and that is how you are going to have a balanced diet. You know that you have got a healthy plan with you when it emphasizes vegetables, fruits, healthy fats, high-quality protein, whole grains, and also legumes. Your plan should also restrict the quantity of excess salt and added sugars in your diet. So, when you are planning your recipes, keep these food groups in mind and then find the recipes suited for your plan.

Also, every group of nutrients is important for your health, and everything has a role to play. Even if you are missing one of these nutrients, they form a gap and affect your health and in extreme cases, can also lead to deficiencies. So, if you want to satisfy your body's needs, make sure you have included each and every food group.

Get Quality Meal Prep Containers

One of the essential tools for starting a meal prep regime is getting quality air-tight containers for yourself. Start checking your cupboard first. If you see that the only things you got are containers with missing lids or those that mismatch in size, then you need to go shopping and get some quality containers. When you don't have the right containers, the process of meal prep can become really very frustrating. So, it is not only worth the money but also will save a lot of your time when you invest in good containers.

But you must also check a few things before you get these containers so that you can be 100% sure that they are perfect for your intended use. If you plan to use them in the dishwasher or freeze or microwave food in them, then these containers should be considered safe for all these purposes. That is also the reason why most people resort to glass containers as they are much safer when you see from the point of view of microwaving and freezing. You can get them online and also in stores near you. They might be a bit costlier than the plastic ones, but they will serve you well.

Your Pantry Should Be Well Stocked

Keeping all the staples in your pantry is essential if you want to meal prep the right way. This will simplify the entire process of creating menus and also streamline the cooking process. Some of the common things that are usually needed are as follows –

- **Legumes** – Garbanzo beans, dried or canned black beans, lentils, pinto beans
- **Whole grains** – polenta, bulgur, oats, quinoa, brown rice
- **Oils** – coconut, avocado, olive, sesame
- **Canned products** – chicken, salmon, tuna, olives, tomatoes, corn, olives
- **Baking goods** – cornstarch, almond flour, coconut flour, baking soda, baking powder

- **Others** – dried fruits, mixed nuts, potatoes, peanut butter, almond butter

Always Keep Enough Spices and Herbs on Hand

One of the things that you need to make your meals taste good are herbs and spices, and they can truly make all the difference to your food. Yes, for some people, having a meal plan that has just enough recipes is sufficient but for those who enjoy the process of cooking or who love their food to be aromatic and full of different spices, using herbs is essential. Spices and herbs are not only flavor-enhancers but they also have a whole lot of health benefits. They can prevent inflammation or even stop cellular damage in certain cases. Some of them also help in keeping blood sugar levels under control.

One such very healthy and useful spice is cinnamon. There is so much that you can do with it, and it also helps in lowering the triglyceride levels in your body and also increases insulin sensitivity and is thus good for those who have higher levels of blood sugar. There are so many dessert recipes that can be made incredibly healthy by the use of cinnamon and you can also add it to sweet potatoes. Another important and important herb is basil which is also known to reduce inflammation. It can be used as a topping in so many veggies and chicken.

Make Time for Meal Planning

If you do not make the process of meal planning and prepping a priority, you will never be successful at it. So, you need to make a conscious choice daily that you are going to set aside some time from your daily routine during which you will plan and, on some days, prep your meals. The time required to plan the meals is not the same for everyone. Some people can do it within fifteen to twenty minutes while some might take an hour in the first few days to figure out what they want to eat and what they should include in their diet plan.

Regardless of the strategy that you are using or the meals that you need to prep, you should always keep some time in your calendar specific to meal planning. People often overlook this aspect and due to their busy schedules, they try to rush the process of planning. What happens is that you don't end up including all the food groups that you should and your meal plan is not balanced. The key to getting good results out of meal planning is not only doing it right but also doing it consistently.

Always Take a Shopping List to the Grocery Store

Once you have figured out the recipes you are going to make this week, it is time for you to make a list of all the ingredients you need and then see what you already have and what things you have to buy. But even after that, you should carry the list to the grocery store along with you. You don't want all of it to go waste just because you missed out one of the key ingredients at the store and also end up buying things that you don't need for the recipes at hand. Having a list on hand will also help you in resisting the temptation of buying all those items which might seem attractive and tasty but are not healthy and definitely not something you need for the upcoming week. Thus, you will save a lot of money in the process as you are buying only what you need.

Depending on the place you live in, you can even find some grocery chains having an online buying option. This means you can simply order what you need from the comforts of your home, and they will deliver everything at your doorstep so that you don't have to go to the store physically. Yes, for this, you might have to pay some extra charge but in some cases, you can get free delivery too especially if your purchasing value is above a certain limit. The best part is that in case of meal planning, you are usually buying in bulk and so the chances are that you will cover the amount needed to avail free delivery services. Also, online shopping of grocery might also give you some special discounts that are specifically meant for online customers and cannot be availed at the store.

Repurpose Leftovers

Repurposing leftovers is a skill that you can learn and put to use, especially if you don't want to cook every day. The process is about cooking a particular man course in extra so that you can use it for lunch or dinner the next day as well. And you don't have to put in extra effort for this. In case you do not like the idea of leftovers, you can always be creative. For example, if you have some leftover chicken from a whole roast, then you can simply repurpose by shredding it and then using it in dishes like soups, tacos or even as salad toppings.

Enjoy the Process

Lastly, I would advise you to enjoy the process of meal prepping because that is the only way in which you can stay consistent at this. Meal prepping is all about building a habit, and if you do not enjoy it, then you will be stuck doing something that you don't love. Once you enjoy the process, it will slowly become a process of self-care as you are meal prepping to eat healthy and thus, stay healthy. It will no longer appear as a task to be done.

In order to make things fun, you can also ask other members of your family to join you. For example, batch cooking soup can be really fun if you do it with others and this also means that you can spend some quality time with your loved ones.

But if you are someone who prefers to do things solo or maybe if you live alone, then play your favorite song or listen to an audiobook that you had planned for a long time and prep your meals. It will be way more fun like that. And before you know it, meal prepping will be a weekend activity that you will look forward to.

Chapter 4:
Easy Meal Prep Recipes

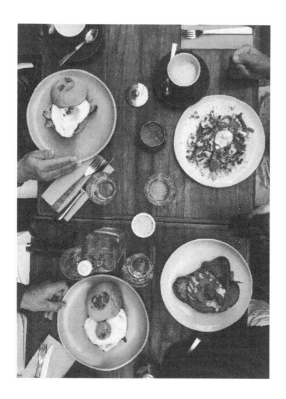

Taking the first step towards a healthy lifestyle is not that difficult, especially with meal prepping. All you need are the right recipes that are not too overwhelming and yet tasty. So this chapter is going to give you a list of ideas for your meal plan.

Breakfast

Mornings are probably the busiest times in every household. If you have kids, then you have to get them ready for school, and if you have to go out for work, then you have to get ready yourself as well. And amidst all that chaos when you can't find what you are looking for or you don't have the time for a shower, you skip on breakfast. Is that healthy? Absolutely not. And so meal prepping can be your ultimate savior. So, here are some breakfast recipes that you should try out.

Freezer Breakfast Sandwiches

Total Prep & Cooking Time: 27 minutes

Yields: 6 servings

Nutrition Facts: Calories: 354 | Protein: 22g | Fat: 16g | Carbs: 27g | Fiber: 1g

Ingredients:

Six each of

- English muffins (cut in half)
- Eggs (large-sized)
- Slices of bacon

- Cheddar cheese slices

To taste: freshly ground pepper and salt

Method:

1. Set the temperature of the oven to 350 degrees and preheat.
2. Now, take a jumbo-sized muffin tin and use cooking spray to coat it. Then take an for each tin and crack the egg in it. Use a fork to whisk the egg lightly. Use pepper and salt to season it. Then take the muffin tin and insert it into the oven. Bake it for about eight to ten minutes. By this time, the egg should be firm. Then, remove the egg from the oven and keep it aside to cool.
3. Take a slice of the bacon and place it on the bottom half of the English muffin and then start layering by adding an egg round and then one slice of cheddar cheese. Lastly, place the other half of the English muffin on top. Use a plastic wrap to seal the sandwich tightly, and then you can set the preparation aside. Use the remaining ingredients to make five more such sandwiches.
4. When you have made all the sandwiches, take a zip-top bag and put all the wrapped sandwiches in it. Before

you seal the bag, press all the air out and transfer the bag to the freezer.

Note: Before eating, simply microwave the sandwich for a minute or two and remember to open one end of the plastic before you heat it so that it does not become soggy.

Oatmeal Breakfast Bites

Total Prep & Cooking Time: 30 minutes

Yields: 24 servings

Nutrition Facts: Calories: 53 | Protein: 2g | Fat: 1g | Carbs: 9g | Fiber: 1g

Ingredients:

Two bananas (ripe, mashed)

Two hundred grams of rolled oats

One beaten egg

Three-quarter cups of milk of your preference

One and a quarter cup of mixed berries (frozen)

One teaspoon of vanilla extract

For greasing: One teaspoon of coconut oil or you can even use butter

Method:

1. Set the temperature of the oven to 350 degrees Fahrenheit and preheat.
2. Take a mixing bowl or large size and then add the oats and mashed bananas into it. In order to ensure that they have fully combined, keep stirring continuously.
3. Add the egg, milk, and vanilla and keep stirring continuously.
4. Then, take the frozen berries and add them too. The berries should be mixed evenly through the mixture. If there are some bigger berries, then you can break them up as well.
5. Now, take a muffin tray and grease it with either butter or coconut oil and then take the mixture and divide it into twenty-four muffin-sized portions.
6. Bake them for about eighteen to twenty minutes until they are ready. A toothpick should come out clean when inserted.

Note: You can keep them in the refrigerator for about four days and three months in the freezer. Simply microwave them for a minute before eating.

Turmeric Scrambled Eggs

Total Prep & Cooking Time: 10 minutes

Yields: 2 servings

Nutrition Facts: Calories: 302 | Protein: 29g | Fat: 18g | Carbs: 6g

Ingredients:

Two tablespoons of milk of your preference

One cup of steamed broccoli

Two teaspoons of turmeric (dried)

Four eggs (large ones)

Eight sausages (small, pre-cooked)

Half a teaspoon of parsley (dried)

To taste: Pepper and salt

Method:

1. Take a small-sized frying pan and coat it with cooking spray. Place it on medium flame.
2. Now, take a small bowl and add the milk, eggs, pepper, salt, parsley, and turmeric. Whisk the mixture well.
3. Once done, pour this mixture into the frying pan. Keep stirring so that you break the eggs and do this for about two to three minutes.
4. Then, flip the eggs with the help of a spatula and then cook them for another two to three minutes or as per your preference.
5. Then, take two meal prep containers and transfer the eggs into them and make sure you divide them properly. Add the sausage and the steamed vegetables too.

Frozen Yogurt Granola Cups

Total Prep & Cooking Time: 3 hours 10 minutes

Yields: 12 servings

Nutrition Facts: Calories: 36 | Protein: 1g | Fat: 1g | Carbs: 4g | Fiber: 1g

Ingredients:

Half a cup each of

- Diced berries of your choice
- Granola

Three-quarter cups of yogurt

Method:

1. Take a muffin pan (mini) and start layering. The granola should be just over half and then, on top of it, divide the berries equally. Then, take one tbsp. of the yogurt and spread on top of the berries in each cup. To remove any air pockets that might have formed, tap the muffin pan a few times on the counter. If there is any granola remaining, you can sprinkle it on top. Then

cover the muffin pan and freeze the preparation for a period of three hours at least.
2. Before you serve the cups, take warm water in a pan and place the bottom of the muffin pan in it. Then to pop out the yogurt bites, use a plastic knife. You can either serve it immediately, or you can put them in ziplock bags and freeze them for later.

Sweet Potato Breakfast Bowl

Total Prep & Cooking Time: 1 hour 20 minutes

Yields: 2 servings

Nutrition Facts: Calories: 356 | Protein: 7g | Fat: 12g | Carbs: 58g | Fiber: 9g

Ingredients:

Sixteen ounces of sweet potatoes

Two tbsps. each of

- Almond butter
- Chopped nuts
- Raisins

To taste: Honey and cinnamon

Method:

1. Set the temperature of the oven to 375 degrees Fahrenheit. Firstly, wash the sweet potatoes nicely and then dry them. Use a fork to poke them multiple times and then use an aluminum foil to wrap them. If you are

using large-sized sweet potatoes, then bake them for about seventy to eighty minutes but if you are using smaller ones, then bake for around sixty minutes. By the end, a fork should easily go into the sweet potato. Before you peel them, set them aside to cool for a minute or two.

2. Once cooled, peel them and make a light mash with honey and cinnamon. You can also use half of a banana and mash it instead of honey.

3. Use chopped nuts and raisins as toppings, or you can use something else as well. Drizzle some amount of almond butter but do this just before serving or reheating.

Choco Chip Oatmeal Squares

Total Prep & Cooking Time: 1 hour

Yields: 12 servings

Nutrition Facts: Calories: 278 | Protein: 5g | Fat: 9g | Carbs: 48g | Fiber: 5g

Ingredients:

Two and a half cups of mashed bananas

Four cups of rolled oats

One cup of mini choco chips (unsweetened)

Three-quarter cups of water

Half a cup of maple syrup

A quarter cup of peanut butter

One teaspoon of salt

Two teaspoons of vanilla extract

Method:

1. Set the temperature of the oven to 350 degrees Fahrenheit and preheat. Take a glass pan and then use parchment paper to line it.
2. Now, take a large-sized bowl and put all the ingredients in it to combine them. So, add the mashed bananas, rolled oats, salt, water, peanut butter, chocolate chips, vanilla extract, and maple syrup and combine all of this properly.
3. Keep mixing until everything is smooth.
4. Now, take the mixture and pour it into a pan that you just lined with parchment paper. Take some additional chocolate chips and sprinkle on top for added flavor.
5. Bake the mixture for about twenty-eight minutes. Firstly, set the timer for twenty minutes. Do not open the door before it. After that, check on the mixture, and if it is not ready yet, then bake for an additional eight minutes.
6. Once done, leave the mixture to cool and then cut into squares.

Bacon Quiche With Potato Crust

Total Prep & Cooking Time: 1 hour

Yields: 4 servings

Nutrition Facts: Calories: 200 | Protein: 16.1g | Fat: 9.5g | Carbs: 14g | Fiber: 2.3g

Ingredients:

Three small-sized gold potatoes (sliced into one-eighth inches)

Cooking spray

Eight ounces of turkey bacon

One red bell pepper (nicely diced)

One tsp. of olive oil

One jalapeno (diced and seeded)

One Roma tomato (large-sized, diced)

Five ounces of organic spinach

Black pepper (freshly ground)

Six eggs

A quarter tsp. of salt

One-third cup of almond milk (unsweetened)

Half a cup of pepper jack cheese (shredded)

Method:

1. Set the oven temperature to 375 degrees Fahrenheit and preheat. Take a pie pan of nine inches and use cooking spray to grease it. Now, take the potato slices and arrange them at the base of the pan and also along the sides. In case you cannot fit them around the sides, don't hesitate to cut some pieces in half. Now, take some more cooking spray and spray on potatoes. Bake the preparation for twenty minutes. After that, remove them from the oven and set them aside to cool for five minutes. Let the oven stay heated.
2. While you are preparing the potato crust, start cooking the turkey bacon. Once they have been cooked, take them out on a plate and keep the plate aside.
3. Now, take the same skillet and add olive oil to it. Add the diced tomatoes, jalapeno, and bell pepper and sauté them for a couple of minutes. After that, add the spinach. Sauté the veggies for a few more minutes. After some time, you will notice that the spinach has

started wilting, and that is when you need to take it down from the heat and set it aside.

4. Take a medium-sized bowl and add the almond milk, eggs, pepper, and salt and whisk them together.
5. Now, take the mixture of veggies and spinach and add them on the crust. Then, take the bacon and place it over the veggies. Season with salt and pepper and sprinkle some shredded cheese on top.
6. Bake the preparation for about thirty-five to forty-five minutes. During this time, the egg will become set and then slowly, puff up to become golden. Then, remove the preparation and cut it into four slices.

Note: If you do not want to use regular potato, then you are free to use sweet potato. In case you want a vegetarian option, just leave the turkey bacon and follow the rest of the steps as they are.

Scrambled Tofu Breakfast Burritos

Total Prep & Cooking Time: 30 minutes

Yields: 4 servings

Nutrition Facts: Calories: 441 | Protein: 16.5g | Fat: 19g | Carbs: 53.5g | Fiber: 8g

Ingredients:

For the tofu,

One teaspoon of oil

Twelve oz. of tofu (extra-firm variety)

Three minces cloves of garlic

Half a cup of freshly chopped parsley

One tablespoon of hummus

Half a teaspoon each of

- Cumin
- Chili powder

One teaspoon of nutritional yeast

A quarter teaspoon of sea salt

Optional – cayenne pepper to taste

For the veggies,

One red bell pepper (medium-sized, thinly sliced)

Five baby potatoes (cut into small pieces)

Half a teaspoon each of

- Chili powder
- Ground cumin

Two cups of kale (chopped)

One teaspoon of oil

Sea salt to taste

Others,

Three to four tortillas (large-sized, gluten-free)

One avocado (medium-sized, ripe, mashed or chopped)

Chunky red salsa

Cilantro

Method:

1. Set the temperature of the oven to 400 degrees Fahrenheit and preheat. Take a baking sheet and then use parchment paper to line it. Also, take a clean towel and use it to wrap the tofu. Then use a cast iron skillet to place on top so that all the excess moisture has been drained out of the tofu. Then, make fine pieces with the help of a fork. Once done, set it aside.
2. Now, add red pepper and potatoes to the baking sheet. Add the spices and drizzle with oil. To ensure that everything has combined well, toss them. Now, bake the mixture for about fifteen to twenty minutes at the end of which they will become brown, and you can use a fork to pierce them easily. In the last five minutes of the baking period, add the kale, add some more seasoning and toss it with the rest of the veggies. The kale will quickly start to wilt.
3. Also, take a large-sized skillet and then place it over medium flame. When the skillet is hot, add oil, tofu, and garlic, and sauté them for seven to ten minutes. After stirring constantly for a few minutes, the tofu will start becoming brown.
4. In the meantime, take a mixing bowl of small size and add the chili powder, hummus, nutritional yeast, cumin, cayenne, and salt and keep stirring so that all the ingredients have combined properly. To form the

sauce, add some water (around one to three tablespoons). Then, take the parsley and add it to the mixture. Keep stirring. Now, take the spice mixture and pour it over the tofu. Keep cooking over medium flame for about three to five minutes. After that, set this mixture aside.

5. Now, it is time for you to assemble the burritos. Take a large-sized tortilla. Firstly, take a generous amount of veggies and add it to the tortilla. After that, take some tofu, cilantro, avocado, and a bit of salsa and add them too. Now, roll the tortilla. Place the seam of the tortilla downwards.

Note: You can refrigerate these for four days.

Avocado Quinoa Frittatas

Total Prep & Cooking Time: 40 minutes

Yields: 12 servings

Nutrition Facts: Calories: 113 | Protein: 4.8g | Fat: 5g | Carbs: 12.6g | Fiber: 2.2g

Ingredients:

Six eggs (large-sized)

One cup of quinoa (uncooked)

Two tbsps. of cilantro (chopped)

One cup of chopped spinach

One avocado (diced, ripe)

One red bell pepper (small-sized, diced)

A quarter cup of red onion (chopped thoroughly)

To taste – black pepper and salt

Optional – half a cup of cheese of your choice (shredded) and one diced jalapeno

Method:

1. Take a small pot and place it on high flame. Pour two cups of water into it. Cook the quinoa. Bring the water to a boil and then cover the pot. After that, bring the flame to a low and continue cooking for fifteen minutes, after which all the water should have been absorbed. Use a fork to fluff the quinoa and then transfer the prepared quinoa to a different bowl where you will leave it to cool for about fifteen minutes.
2. In the meantime, set the temperature of the oven to 350 degrees Fahrenheit and preheat. Take a muffin pan of twelve cups and spray each liner with cooking spray generously.
3. Take a large-sized bowl and in it, add the eggs and whisk them nicely. Add the onion, veggies, avocado, pepper, and salt and you can also add the cheese and jalapeno if you are using them. Also, take the cooled quinoa and add it.
4. Now, take the muffin pan and divide the mixture evenly into each of these cups. Bake the preparation for about twenty to twenty-five minutes. By this time, the eggs will be set, and the edges will have started to become a bit golden brownish.
5. Now, take the pan and let it cool for about five to ten minutes. You can store these in the container and then

keep them in the refrigerator for about five to seven days.

Note: Make sure you line the muffin liners properly; others, the frittatas, won't turn out to be so good because they tend to stick. The nutrition measures mentioned here do not include the cheese. So, if you are indeed using the cheese, then the calorie value will have to be increased by fifteen calories or even more. You can veggies of your choice and not stay limited to these. You can add mushrooms sweet potatoes, or even zucchinis.

Lunch

Planning your meals ahead of time means that you are going to get homemade meals for lunch that assures a balanced diet. And, you can also keep your taste buds happy if you select the recipes wisely. Here are some ideas for you.

Sweet and Spicy Tempeh Bowls

Total Prep & Cooking Time: 30 minutes

Yields: 4 servings

Nutrition Facts: Calories: 667 | Protein: 26g | Fat: 33g | Carbs: 68g | Fiber: 12g

Ingredients:

For the sweet and spicy tempeh,

Eight ounces of tempeh

Half a teaspoon each of

- Salt
- Cayenne pepper
- Smoked paprika
- Garlic powder

Half a cup of water

One tablespoon of olive oil

Two tablespoons of brown sugar

For polenta,

Three cups of water

One cup of cornmeal

Two tablespoons of butter

Half a teaspoon of salt

For bowl toppings,

Two ounces of cheddar cheese (shredded)

Fifteen ounces of rinsed black beans

Two sliced green onions (large-sized)

One avocado (thinly sliced)

Four tablespoons of ranch dressing

Method:

1. Start with the preparation of the tempeh and cutting it into thin triangles of about thirty-two in number. Once done, take a large-sized skillet, and it should be non-stick and then add the tempeh triangles in it.
2. Now, it is time for you to make the spicy and sweet marinade. Take garlic powder, water, olive oil, brown sugar, salt, cayenne, and smoked paprika and mix them together. Once done, take this mixture and add it to the tempeh. Place the skillet on medium-high and then keep stirring from time to time as you simmer the tempeh. Continue doing this until you notice that all the liquid has evaporated. In about ten minutes or so, you will notice that there is a slight browning of the tempeh, and that is when you have to remove it from the heat.
3. Now, it is time to make the polenta. Take a saucepot of medium size and in it, add salt, water, and cornmeal and combine them together. Then, take the pot and place it on medium-high flame. Keep whisking and bring it to a boil. Once it is boiling, turn down the flame to a medium-low and let it be like that for two to three minutes. The polenta will gradually thicken. Once done, remove it from the flame, add the butter, and stir it in nicely.

4. Now, it is time to make the bowls. First, take a cup of polenta and then a quarter of the spicy and sweet tempeh triangles. After that, take a quarter of the black beans that you had rinsed and about half an ounce of cheddar cheese (shredded) and place them in the bowl. Add a quarter portion of the avocado and sprinkle some of the chopped green onions on top. Then, drizzle some of the ranch dressing. You can either serve immediately or even refrigerate it for later.

Vegetable Barley Soup

Total Prep & Cooking Time: 55 minutes

Yields: 6 servings (two cups for each)

Nutrition Facts: Calories: 277| Protein: 7.4g | Fat: 6g | Carbs: 53g | Fiber: 9.1g

Ingredients:

Two garlic cloves

One large-sized yellow onion

Half a pound of carrots

Two tablespoons of olive oil

Half a teaspoon each of

- Dried oregano
- Basil

A cup each of

- Pearled barley
- Frozen green beans

One russet potato

Twenty-eight ounces of tomatoes (diced)

Six cups of vegetable broth

A pinch of black pepper (freshly cracked)

Half a cup each of

- Frozen peas
- Frozen corn

One tablespoon of lemon juice

For garnishing: fresh parsley (almost a handful)

Method:

1. Start by mincing the garlic and dicing the onion. Now, take a large-sized soup pot and add the olive oil, garlic, and onion to it. Place the pot over medium and sauté the onion and garlic. Do it until they become transparent and soft, and this will take about five minutes.
2. At the same time, peel the carrots and then dice them. When the onions have become soft, take the carrots and add them to the pot as well. Add the diced tomatoes too. Then add basil, barley, pepper, oregano, and the vegetable broth.

3. Keep stirring continuously so that everything has combined well. Then, place the lid on the pot and turn the flame up to medium-high and bring it to a boil. Once the soup starts to boil, turn down the flame and bring it to a simmer. Don't open the lid although stir the soup occasionally. Let it cook for half an hour.
4. While the soup is simmering, take the potato, peel it and then dice into cubes of half an inch. Once the barley is soft and tender, take the potatoes and add them to the soup. Cook it for about ten more minutes.
5. When the potatoes have become tender, take the frozen corn, green beans, and peas and add them to the pot. Keep stirring so that everything combines well. Keep the pot on the flame for five more minutes, and finally, pour in the lemon juice. Combine it by stirring.
6. Taste the soup and if need be, then adjust the pepper and salt accordingly. If you want to garnish it, then add parsley on top.

Roasted Vegetables and Sausage

Total Prep & Cooking Time: 55 minutes

Yields: 4 servings

Nutrition Facts: Calories: 660 | Protein: 17.6g | Fat: 43g | Carbs: 50g | Fiber: 4.3g

Ingredients:

For the smoky vinaigrette,

Two tablespoons of red wine vinegar

A quarter cup of olive oil

A quarter teaspoon each of

- Salt
- Dried oregano
- Garlic powder
- Sugar

Half a teaspoon of smoked paprika

One teaspoon of Dijon mustard

A little bit of black pepper (freshly cracked)

For the veggies and sausage,

One pound of broccoli

Twelve ounces of smoked sausage

One red onion

One bell pepper of your choice

For serving,

Freshly chopped parsley

A cup of uncooked white rice (long-grained)

Method:

1. Set the temperature of the oven to 400 degrees Fahrenheit and preheat. Use parchment paper to line a baking sheet.
2. Take a small-sized bowl and add the ingredients of the vinaigrette to it, that is, the red wine vinegar, olive oil, dried oregano, garlic powder, Dijon mustard, smoked paprika, dried oregano, pepper, salt, and sugar. In order to mix them properly, whisk the ingredients together, or if you are using a jar, then close and shake it thoroughly. Once done, set it aside.

3. Take a smoked sausage and slice it into medallions of half an inch. Take the broccoli and cut it into bite-sized florets. Prepare the bell pepper and onion by dicing them too. Then, place all of these veggies and the sausage on the baking sheet and arrange them properly.
4. Take two tablespoons of the vinaigrette and spread it over the veggies and sausage. Toss them so that they get coated evenly.
5. Now, put the baking sheet into the preheated oven and roast the preparation for about thirty-five to forty minutes. By the end, you will notice that the edges have browned. Halfway through, stir the veggies a bit.
6. While you are roasting the veggies and the sausage, prepare the rice. Take a saucepot and add two cups of water to cook the rice. Cover the pot and bring the water to a boil. Keep the flame on high, but after boiling turn the flame to medium-low again. Let the water simmer for about fifteen minutes. After that, turn off the flame and keep the pot as it is without disturbing it for five minutes. Before serving, use a fork to fluff the rice.
7. Once the vegetables and sausage have finished roasting, take the remaining preparation of vinaigrette and add it. Toss the veggies and sausages properly so

that they get evenly coated. Add a pinch of pepper and salt if it is needed.

8. Each container should have a quarter cup of rice and a quarter portion of the sausages and veggies. Drizzle some vinaigrette on top and some freshly chopped parsley as well.

Jerk Chicken With Black Beans and Pineapple Salsa

Total Prep & Cooking Time: 45 minutes

Yields: 4 servings

Nutrition Facts: Calories: 298 | Protein: 24.6g | Fat: 5.8g | Carbs: 55g | Fiber: 9g

Ingredients:

Four cups of rice (cooked)

For the jerk chicken,

Two chicken breasts (boneless, skinless)

One tablespoon of cooking oil

One tablespoon of jerk seasoning

For the black bean and pineapple salsa,

Fifteen ounces of well-rinsed black beans

Two cups of fresh pineapple tidbits

Half a cup of cilantro (coarsely chopped)

One-third cup of red onion (finely diced)

A quarter teaspoon of salt

One lime

Optional – red pepper flakes (only a pinch)

Method:

1. Start by cooking the rice first. Once your rice is cooked, cool it, and then divide it into the meal prep containers equally.
2. Prepare the black bean pineapple salsa while you are cooking the rice. First, take the pineapple tidbits and chop them coarsely so that the size of the pieces is similar to that of the black beans. Now, take a large-sized bowl and add the chopped cilantro, diced red onion, black beans, and chopped pineapple to it.
3. On top of all these ingredients, squeeze the juice out of one lime. Also, add a few red pepper flakes if you want and a quarter teaspoon of salt, which is mandatory. Now, mix all the ingredients together by stirring and then taste to see if everything is okay.
4. The next step is to start with the jerk chicken. Firstly, use a paper towel to pat the chicken dry. Then, you need to pound the chicken breasts, but we do not want

any splatter so what we will do is that we will cover the breasts with a plastic wrap and then use a rolling pin to pound them evenly. Once done, take the jerk seasoning and sprinkle it properly on both sides of the pounded chicken breasts and then to coat them well, use your hands to rub the seasoning.

5. Now, take a large skillet and add cooking oil to it. Once the oil is hot, take the chicken breasts and add them to the skillet. You have to make both sides of the chicken cook evenly and get a nice brown coating. There should no pink portions, even at the center of the chicken. It will take you almost seven minutes on each side of the chicken. If you want to be extra safe and you have a meat thermometer, then check whether the internal temperature has reached 165 degrees Fahrenheit.

6. Then, take a clean cutting board and transfer the chicken to it. Let it cool for five minutes and then start slicing then into wide strips of half an inch.

7. Top the rice in the meal prep containers with the black bean pineapple salsa and then place a few strips of the jerk chicken. If there is any lime remaining, then slice it into wedges and place it on top, or you can even sprinkle some fresh juice before eating.

Black-Eyed Peas Meal Prep

This recipe requires you to make two things – sweet potato cornbread and black-eyed peas, and so I have explained both separately.

Sweet Potato Cornbread

Total Prep & Cooking Time: 55 minutes

Yields: 8 servings

Nutrition Facts: Calories: 277 | Protein: 6g | Fat: 13.8g | Carbs: 33g | Fiber: 3.3g

Ingredients:

One sweet potato (medium-sized)

One cup of all-purpose flour

One and a half cups of yellow cornmeal

Half a cup each of

- Sugar

- Sour cream

One teaspoon of salt

One tablespoon of baking powder

Half a teaspoon each of

- Nutmeg
- Cinnamon

Two tablespoons of canola oil

Two eggs (large-sized)

Three-quarter cups of milk

For the skillet: Half a tablespoon of canola oil

Method:

1. Start by peeling the sweet potatoes. Then, cut them into small pieces of one inch. Then take a pot, add the diced potatoes in it, and then pour water so that the potatoes are all covered. Cover the pot. Turn the flame to high and boil the potatoes. Once done, they should fall apart with the help of a fork. This should be done by ten minutes or so. Once all the potatoes are tender, drain them and keep them aside.
2. Take an iron skillet and coat it with oil. Set the temperature of the oven to 425 degrees Fahrenheit and keep the skillet inside. Preheat.

3. Take a large-sized bowl and in it, add flour, cornmeal, salt, baking powder, sugar, nutmeg, and cinnamon and stir until everything has properly mixed.
4. Now, take the drained potatoes and mash them. Make sure that they have become smooth. Take one and a half cups of those mashed potatoes and then transfer them to a large-sized bowl. Add the milk, sour cream, and also two tablespoons of oil. Keep whisking until thoroughly combined. Now, add the eggs too and whisk the mixture again.
5. Take this mixture of sweet potatoes and add them to the dry ingredients that you had kept in a separate bowl. Keep stirring. Make sure that no dry mix should be present in the corners of the bowl. Don't over-mix. It is okay to have small lumps in the mixture.
6. Now, open the preheated oven and take the hot skillet out. Scoop out the batter and pour it into the skillet. Even out the top of the batter and then return the skillet into the oven. Bake the mixture for about twenty-five minutes. The center will become golden brown and puffed. The edges will seem slightly cracked too. Once done, remove it from the oven and then let it cool a bit. After that, slice it into eight pieces.

Black-Eyed Peas

Total Prep & Cooking Time: 10 hours

Yields: 5 servings

Nutrition Facts: Calories: 369 | Protein: 27g | Fat: 17g | Carbs: 31g | Fiber: 11g

Ingredients:

Two tablespoons of olive oil

One pound of dry black-eyed peas

A quarter teaspoon of cayenne pepper

Half a tablespoon of smoked paprika

One teaspoon of oregano

Half a bunch of celery

Three garlic cloves

One onion

One bay leaf

A pinch of pepper (freshly cracked)

Twelve ounces of fresh greens (kale or collard greens)

Six cups of vegetable broth

Method:

1. You have to start this recipe the night before and take large a container filled with cool water in which you can soak the black-eyed peas. The water in the bowl should be at least three times the amount of peas. Keep the bowl in the refrigerator overnight while the peas are soaking.
2. The next day, when you are ready to cook, take a large pot and olive oil to it. Mince the garlic, dice the onion, and cut the celery into slices. Add all of these to the pot and place the pot on medium flame. Sauté the ingredients, and after a while, you will notice that the onions that have become translucent.
3. Now take a colander and drain the peas. Use cool water to rinse the peas. Add these peas to the pot after rinsing where you sautéed the vegetables. Also, add the smoked paprika, oregano, pepper, and cayenne pepper. Add the vegetable broth and bay leaf too. Combine them well by stirring.
4. Cover the pot with a lid. Turn up the flame and let the soup boil. Once it starts to boil, lower the flame. Let it simmer for an hour.

5. After that, the black-eyed peas will become soft and tender. Then, take the greens and add them to the pot. After stirring for a while, they will become wilted. Take a spatula to smash some of the peas in the pot. This will help in thickening the liquid.
6. Now, turn the flame again to medium and let it simmer. Cook without a lid for about half an hour. The liquid should have thickened even more. Taste the dish and then adjust the salt accordingly.

Note: Once you have prepared both and divided into 5 meal-prep containers, you will have 3 cornbread as leftovers. You can freeze them for later.

Dinner

When you return home tired from work, no one likes to prepare food, and so meal prepping can definitely lift off a lot of stress from your shoulders. So, here are some easy dinner recipes that you can prepare in advance.

Honey Glazed Meatballs

Total Prep & Cooking Time: 55 minutes

Yields: 8 servings (5 meatballs for each)

Nutrition Facts: Calories: 295| Protein: 27g | Fat: 11g | Carbs: 18.6g | Fiber: 1.4g

Ingredients:

For the meatballs,

One cup of panko breadcrumbs (whole-wheat variety)

Two pounds of lean ground turkey

Half a teaspoon each of

- Salt

- Garlic powder
- Black pepper

A quarter cup of chopped green onions

Two eggs

For the sauce,

One tablespoon of ginger (freshly grated)

Three tablespoons each of

- Honey
- Rice vinegar
- Soy sauce (reduced sodium variety)

Three minced cloves of garlic

A quarter cup of Sriracha

Half a teaspoon of sesame oil (toasted)

Method:

1. Set the temperature of the oven to 375 degrees Fahrenheit and preheat.
2. Take a large-sized mixing bowl and in it, add the breadcrumbs, ground turkey, green onions, eggs,

pepper, salt, and garlic and keep mixing until everything has properly combined. Then, take the mixture and form balls of one and a half inches each. There will be roughly forty balls from the mixture. Now, take prepared baking sheets and place the balls on them separately. The sheets should be sprayed by cooking spray.

3. Now, bake the meatballs for a period of twenty to twenty-five minutes until they are fully cooked or have browned.

4. Take a small-sized saucepan and start preparing the sauce while the meatballs are baking. Combine all the ingredients in it. Then place it over medium flame and bring it to a boil. Keep whisking from time to time. After that, reduce the flame. Let it simmer for ten minutes, and gradually you will see that the sauce has started thickening in consistency. Once done, toss the sauce with the meatballs.

Note: You can serve this preparation or freeze in meal prep containers along with some brown rice.

Soy Glazed Chicken With Garlic Noodles

This recipe requires you to make two things – garlic noodles and soy-glazed chicken, and so I have explained both separately.

Garlic Noodles

Total Prep & Cooking Time: 25 minutes

Yields: 4 servings

Nutrition Facts: Calories: 304 | Protein: 15g | Fat: 20g | Carbs: 88g | Fiber: 3g

Ingredients:

Four garlic cloves

Eight ounces of pasta (angel hair)

Four tablespoons of butter

Half a bunch of green onions

Two tablespoons each of

- Oyster sauce
- Brown sugar

One teaspoon of sesame oil

Two teaspoons of soy sauce

Method:

1. Firstly, take a bowl and add the brown sugar, oyster sauce, sesame oil, and soy sauce to it. Then, keep stirring until all the ingredients have fully combined.
2. Now, take a large pot of water and place it over a high flame. Bring the water to a boil. Follow the directions mentioned in the package to cook the noodles. This will take about seven to ten minutes. Then, take a colander and drain the noodles. Keep them aside.
3. While the noodles are cooking, start slicing the green onions and also mince the garlic. Take a large-sized skillet and put it over medium flame. Melt the butter in it. Once the butter has become bubbly, add the onions and the garlic. Save a bit of onion for garnishing and then keep sautéing for two minutes until the noodles are nicely fragrant.
4. Then, take the skillet off from the flame. Add the mixture of oyster sauce along with the drained pasta into the skillet. In order to make sure that the pasta has fully coated, keep stirring. In case you are finding it

difficult to stir the pasts because it has become sticky, you should add some hot water into the skillet, and the pasta will loosen up. Once done, garnish with the green onions that you had set aside.

Soy Glazed Chicken

Total Prep & Cooking Time: 1 hour

Yields: 4 servings

Nutrition Facts: Calories: 467 | Protein: 29g | Fat: 35g | Carbs: 8g | Fiber: 1g

Ingredients:

For the marinade,

One-eighth cup of brown sugar

Half a tablespoon of freshly grated ginger

One and a half tablespoons of soy sauce

One clove of garlic

Half a tablespoon of cooking oil

A pinch of pepper (freshly cracked)

For the chicken,

Four chicken thighs (skinless, boneless)

A quarter tablespoon of cooking oil

For the garnishes,

Half a teaspoon of sesame seeds

One green onion

Method:

1. Grate the ginger and then mince the garlic using a box grater. Take a small-sized bowl and add the soy sauce, brown sugar, pepper, ginger, garlic, and cooking oil in it. Keep stirring. Now, take the chicken in a shallow dish and pour the marinade you made over the chicken. Turn the chicken pieces so that all of them are coated with the marinade. Keep the marinated chicken in the refrigerator for at least thirty minutes, or you can keep it for a day as well.
2. When the chicken is ready, place a large-sized skillet on medium heat. Then, add the cooking oil in it. Ensure that the entire bottom of the skillet is covered with the oil. Then, add in the chicken pieces and cook them

through so that they are browned evenly. Take the chicken out and place it on a clean plate.

3. After removing the chicken, take the leftover marinade and add it to the skillet. Let it boil. Also, whisk the marinade so that if anything has been left on the walls of the skillet will be mixed with the marinade. Let it boil, and within a few minutes, it will form a thick and browned glaze. So, turn the flame off and add the chicken into the skillet again. Coat the thick glaze onto the chicken pieces nicely and use sesame seeds and green onion slices for garnishing.

Note: Prepare the containers by adding the noodles and soy-glazed chicken after dividing them into four equal parts. In one part of the container, keep some steamed broccoli too. Divide three-quarter pounds of broccoli florets into four containers.

Beef and Broccoli

Total Prep & Cooking Time: 30 minutes

Yields: 4 servings

Nutrition Facts: Calories: 191 | Protein: 19g | Fat: 9g | Carbs: 6g | Fiber: 1g

Ingredients:

Three-quarter pounds of sirloin or flank steak (fat should be trimmed, sliced)

Two minced cloves of garlic

Water (required for blanching broccoli)

One tbsp. of cooking oil

A quarter tsp. of ginger (freshly grated)

Three and a half cup of broccoli florets

For the beef marinade,

One tsp. each of

- Soy sauce (low-sodium variety)

- Arrowroot or cornstarch

Half a tsp. of sesame oil (toasted)

One-eighth tsp. of pepper

Optional – a quarter tsp. of dark soy sauce (it gives added flavor and color)

For the sauce,

One and a half tsps. of soy sauce (low-sodium variety)

One and a half tbsps. of oyster sauce

Two tsps. each of

- Cornstarch
- Granulated sugar

One-third cup of chicken broth

Half a tsp. of dry sherry (optional)

One tsp. of sesame oil (toasted)

To taste – pepper and salt

For serving – quinoa, brown rice or noodles

Method:

1. Start by marinating the beef. Take all the required ingredients in one bowl and then mix them properly. Then, pour in the beef slices. Keep stirring until everything is evenly coated. Set this aside for a period of at least ten minutes.
2. Meanwhile, you can take the broccoli and blanch it. Take a wok or non-stick sauté pan and put it on high flame. Boil water in it. Then, add the florets of broccoli and cook them for about thirty seconds. Then, carefully drain the water and right after that, rinse the broccoli with cold water so that the cooking process is stopped. Keep it aside. You can skip this step in case you are not blanching the broccoli.
3. Now, make the sauce. Take all the ingredients required in a small-sized bowl. Mix them and keep it aside.
4. Now, take a pan and heat cooking oil in it for about two minutes. You can use the same pan you used for blanching the broccoli. Before you add anything to the pan, it should be hot enough so that you see a bit of smoke rising.
5. Then, add the beef to the pan. Make sure that you have spread all the pieces so that they do not lie over one another and are present in a single layer. Sear the pieces until they turn brown. Then, add the garlic and keep cooking the beef so that there is no pink portion

in it. But don't overcook it. It should take you only a couple of minutes more.

6. After that, add the sauce and keep stirring. Gradually, the sauce will start boiling and then start to thicken. Stir for about thirty seconds. Then, if you need to thin the sauce out, add some water.

7. Add the broccoli quickly, and now you need to toss everything thoroughly so that they are all coated with the sauce. Add pepper and salt to taste.

8. Sprinkle some green onions and sesame seeds on top if you want.

BBQ Baked Zucchini and Salmon

Total Prep & Cooking Time: 30 minutes

Yields: 4 servings

Nutrition Facts: Calories: 407 | Protein: 35g | Fat: 14.4g | Carbs: 36g | Fiber: 5.3g

Ingredients:

For the salmon,

Half a cup of BBQ sauce (gluten-free)

Ten to twelve oz. of salmon fillets

One tablespoon each of

- Honey
- Apple cider vinegar

A quarter teaspoon of black pepper

A pinch of kosher salt

One teaspoon of garlic (minced)

For meal prep,

Three cups of cauliflower rice or one cup of uncooked quinoa

A pinch of sea salt

Two cups of broth (needed for cooking quinoa)

One tablespoon of olive oil

A bunch of cilantro (nicely chopped)

Two zucchini (medium-sized, spiralized)

One oz. of pumpkin seeds

Lime wedges or lime

One medium-sized avocado (sliced)

To taste – pepper and kosher salt

Method:

For the salmon,

1. Set the temperature of the oven to 400 degrees Fahrenheit and then preheat. Also, take a baking sheet and use a foil to line it properly. Once done, keep it aside.
2. Take a small-sized bowl, and add the BBQ sauce in it along with the other ingredients as well. Mix them.

3. Now, take two tablespoons of this mixture and spread it on each fillet of salmon.
4. Bake the salmon for about ten to twelve minutes. Then, broil the preparation for about two minutes until you notice that edges of the salmon to start browning. But you should check after the eight-minute mark to prevent yourself from overcooking the salmon. Then, sprinkle a pinch of salt over the salmon.
5. Use a fork to break the salmon.

For meal prep,

1. Cook the quinoa based on the instructions given in the package. Cook it until it becomes fluffy.
2. Take one-third cup of cooked quinoa into each meal-prep container. Then, add three oz. of BBQ salmon on top of it.
3. Then, take a scoop of zucchini noodles and place them in another compartment of the container and then add a few pumpkin seeds on top.
4. To garnish, add a splash of lemon or juice of lime wedges, cilantro, and slices of avocado. Add pepper and salt based on taste.
5. If you want, you can even brush a bit of extra BBQ sauce on top of the fillets.

Thai Coconut Quinoa Bowls

Total Prep & Cooking Time: 45 minutes

Yields: 4 servings

Nutrition Facts: Calories: 250 | Protein: 8g | Fat: 16g | Carbs: 19g | Fiber: 6g

Ingredients:

For roasted sweet potatoes,

Two tbsps. of olive oil

Two sweet potatoes (large-sized, cubed)

One-eighth tsp. each of

- Freshly ground pepper
- Salt

One tbsp. of garlic (minced)

One tsp. of black sesame seeds

For the coconut quinoa,

Fifteen ounces of coconut milk

One cup of quinoa (uncooked)

One tbsp. of maple syrup

Half a cup of water

For the purple cabbage slaw,

One carrot (large-sized, sliced into thin sticks)

One red pepper (large-sized, sliced)

One cup each of

- Shelled edamame
- Sliced purple cabbage

One tsp. each of

- Ginger (freshly grated)
- Soy sauce

One tbsp. each of

- Fresh lime juice
- Apple cider vinegar
- Olive oil

One-eighth tsp. of salt

For the peanut sauce,

Two and a half tbsps. each of

- Water
- Peanut butter (all-natural)

One tsp. each of

- Maple syrup
- Soy sauce

For toppings,

Juice of one lime

A quarter cup each of

- Chopped peanuts
- Freshly chopped cilantro

Black sesame seeds

Method:

For the coconut quinoa,

1. Take a medium-sized pot and add all the ingredients in it. Place the pot over medium flame and then bring it to a boil.
2. When the boiling starts, reduce the flame to low. Keep it covered and reduce it to a simmer. Let it be like that for twenty minutes or so. By then, all the liquid will be absorbed, and the quinoa will be fully cooked.

For the roasted sweet potatoes,

1. Set the temperature of the oven to 400 degrees Fahrenheit and preheat. Take a large-sized baking sheet and drizzle olive oil on it after arranging the sweet potatoes. Toss them so that they are fully coated with the oil.
2. Use salt, minced garlic, and pepper to season the potatoes. Sprinkle some black sesame seeds as well. Toss them again.
3. Roast the potatoes for about half an hour.

For the purple cabbage slaw,

1. Take a bowl and add the edamame, purple cabbage, red pepper, and carrot to it. Mix them and set the bowl aside.
2. Now, make the dressing. Take another bowl and in it, add apple cider vinegar, olive oil, soy sauce, lime juice, grated ginger, maple syrup, and salt and whisk them together.
3. Toss the veggies thoroughly in the dressing to coat them evenly. Set the preparation aside.

For the peanut sauce,

Take a jar or medium-sized bowl and add all the peanut sauce ingredients to it. Mix all the ingredients so that all of them combine well.

For assembly,

1. First, distribute the coconut quinoa evenly into the meal prep containers. Then take the coleslaw and the sweet potatoes and divide them too.
2. If you are eating it immediately, then drizzle some peanut sauce on top and add lime wedges, chopped cilantro, chopped peanuts, and some more black sesame seeds.

Salads and Vegetables

Vegetables and greens are always important for your diet because of the immense amount of vitamins, minerals, and antioxidants they provide and so here are some salads and vegetable recipes that you can easily meal prep with things available at every grocery store.

Artichoke and Avocado Pasta Salad

Total Prep & Cooking Time: 30 minutes

Yields: 10 servings

Nutrition Facts: Calories: 188 | Protein: 6g | Fat: 10g | Carbs: 21g | Fiber: 2g

Ingredients:

Two cups of spiral pasta (uncooked)

A quarter cup of Romano cheese (grated)

One can (fourteen oz.) of artichoke hearts (coarsely chopped and drained well)

One avocado (medium-sized, ripe, cubed)

Two plum tomatoes (chopped coarsely)

For the dressing,

One tbsp. of fresh cilantro (chopped)

Two tbsps. of lime juice

A quarter cup of canola oil

One and a half tsps. of lime zest (grated)

Half a tsp. each of

- Pepper (freshly ground)
- Kosher salt

Method:

1. Follow the directions mentioned on the package for cooking the pasta. Drain them well and rinse using cold water.
2. Then, take a large-sized bowl and in it, add the pasta along with the tomatoes, artichoke hearts, cheese, and avocado. Combine them well. Then, take another bowl and add all the ingredients of the dressing in it. Whisk them together and, once combined, add the dressing over the pasta.
3. Gently toss the mixture to coat everything evenly in the dressing and then refrigerate.

Apple Arugula and Turkey Salad in a Jar

Total Prep & Cooking Time: 20 minutes

Yields: 4 servings

Nutrition Facts: Calories: 471 | Protein: 45g | Fat: 19g | Carbs: 33g | Fiber: 5g

Ingredients:

Three tbsps. of red wine vinegar

Two tbsps. of chives (freshly minced)

Half a cup of orange juice

One to three tbsps. of sesame oil

A quarter tsp. each of

- Pepper (coarsely ground)
- Salt

For the salad,

Four tsps. of curry powder

Four cups each of

- Turkey (cubed, cooked)
- Baby spinach or fresh arugula

A quarter tsp. of salt

Half a tsp. of pepper (coarsely ground)

One cup of halved green grapes

One apple (large-sized, chopped)

Eleven oz. of mandarin oranges (properly drained)

One tbsp. of lemon juice

Half a cup each of

- Walnuts (chopped)
- Dried cranberries or pomegranate seeds

Method:

1. Take a small-sized bowl and, in it, add the first 6 ingredients from the list into it. Whisk them. Then take a large bowl and in it, add the turkey and then add the seasonings on top of it. Toss the turkey cubes to coat them with the seasoning. Take another bowl and in it, add the lemon juice and toss the apple chunks in the juice.

2. Take four jars and divide the layers in the order I mention here - first goes the orange juice mixture, the second layer is that of the turkey, then apple, oranges, grapes, cranberries or pomegranate seeds, walnuts, and spinach or arugula. Cover the jars and then refrigerate them.

Summertime Slaw

Total Prep & Cooking Time: 50 minutes

Yields: 10-12 servings

Nutrition Facts: Calories: 138 | Protein: 1g | Fat: 6g | Carbs: 21g | Fiber: 2g

Ingredients:

One-third cup of canola oil

Three-quarter cups each of

- White vinegar
- Sugar

One tsp. each of

- Pepper
- Salt

One tbsp. of water

Half a tsp. of red pepper flakes (crushed and optional)

Two tomatoes (medium-sized, seeded, peeled, and chopped)

One pack of coleslaw mix (fourteen oz.)

One sweet red pepper (small-sized, chopped)

One green pepper (small-sized, chopped)

One onion (large-sized, chopped)

Half a cup of sweet pickle relish

Method:

1. Take a saucepan of large size and in it, combine water, sugar, oil, vinegar, pepper, salt, and if you want, then red pepper flakes too. Cook them over medium heat by continuously stirring the mixture. Keep stirring until it comes to a boil. Cook for another two minutes or so and make sure that all the sugar has dissolved. Once done, cool the mixture to room temperature by stirring it.
2. Take a salad bowl of large size and in it, combine the pickle relish, coleslaw mix, peppers, onion, and tomatoes. On top of the mixture, add the dressing and toss the mixture to coat it properly. Cover the mixture and put it in the refrigerator for a night.

Zucchini and Tomato Spaghetti

Total Prep & Cooking Time: 30 minutes

Yields: 4 servings

Nutrition Facts: Calories: 330 | Protein: 7.1g | Fat: 20g | Carbs: 35.3g | Fiber: 8g

Ingredients:

Two large-sized zucchini nicely sprialized

Three cups of red and yellow cherry tomatoes

Four oz. of spaghetti (whole wheat – optional)

Toppings – grated parmesan

For the avocado sauce,

A quarter cup of olive oil

One avocado

Half a cup of parsley (fresh)

Half a tsp. of salt

Three-four green onions (only the green parts)

One lemon (juiced)

One clove of garlic

A pinch of pepper (freshly ground)

Method:

1. Firstly, take all the ingredients of the sauce and pulse them so that they are combined well and form a smooth mixture. Set it aside.
2. Then, follow the directions mentioned in the package for cooking the spaghetti. Drain the cooked spaghetti and keep it aside too.
3. Take a large-sized skillet and heat the cherry tomatoes in it. Use a bit of olive oil. Keep cooking the tomatoes until they seem well-roasted, and they will also seem loosened with their skins split. Once done, remove the tomatoes from the flame and set it aside.
4. Then, add the zucchini to the same skillet. Stir and toss them for about two minutes until they look crisp. Then, add the avocado sauce and the spaghetti. Keep tossing until everything has properly combined. Season with pepper and salt as per taste. Top with parmesan and the tomatoes that you had reserved earlier.

Note: If you want to make this super-healthy, you can stick only to the zucchini and skip the pasta altogether. When the tomatoes are cooking, keep the lid covered because the hot oil tends to splatter.

White Bean Salad

Total Prep & Cooking Time: 10 minutes

Yields: 4 servings

Nutrition Facts: Calories: 449 | Protein: 23.6g | Fat: 23.3g | Carbs: 39.7g

Ingredients:

For the salad,

Two green peppers coarsely chopped

Half a cup each of

- Chopped cucumber
- Chopped tomatoes

One and a half cups of white beans (boiled)

A quarter cup each of

- Green onions (chopped)
- Fresh dill (chopped)
- Parsley (chopped)

Four eggs (hard-boiled)

For the dressing,

One tbsp. of lemon juice

One tsp. of vinegar

Two tbsps. of olive oil

One tsp. of sumac

Half a tsp. of salt

For quick onion pickle,

One tsp. each of

- Sumac
- Salt
- Vinegar

One tbsp. of lemon juice

Two thinly sliced red onions (medium-sized)

Two cups of water (hot)

Method:

1. Take a large-sized bowl and add all the salad ingredients in it, but keep the eggs aside.
2. In case you do not want to pickle the onions, you can simply make thin slices and then mix them with the

other ingredients. But, if you do want to pickle the onions, then continue with it before you move on to the dressing. The recipe for the onions is mentioned later.

3. Take all the ingredients of the dressing together in one bowl and whisk them together. Then, drizzle the dressing over the salad. Toss well, and on the top, place halved eggs.

For the pickled onions,

1. First, take very hot water and place the sliced onions in it. Blanch the onions for one minute and then immediately transfer them into a pot of very cold water so that the cooking stops. Let them stay in that pot of cold water for a few minutes. Once done, drain them well.
2. Mix sumac, lemon juice, salt, and vinegar together and then pour the mixture over the onion that you just drained. Keep it for five to ten minutes.
3. Then, add the onions into the mixture of salad and stir well. Keep some onions aside so that you can use them as a topping.

Lentil Bolognese

Total Prep & Cooking Time: 60 minutes

Yields: 4-6 servings

Nutrition Facts: Calories: 486 | Protein: 29.3g | Fat: 9g | Carbs: 78.2g | Fiber: 15g

Ingredients:

Two boxes of penne pasta

One onion (medium-sized, finely chopped)

One red bell pepper (finely chopped)

Two tbsps. of olive oil

Two carrots (large-sized, sliced)

Four cloves of garlic (large ones, minced)

One tbsp. of miso

One tsp. each of

- Pepper
- Salt

Four cups of water

One can of tomato paste (measuring five and a half ounces)

One cup each of

- Brown lentils (dried)
- Cherry tomatoes (halved)

Toppings (optional) – black pepper, sage leaves, parmesan (grated)

Method:

1. Take a large-sized skillet and start by heating the oil in it on medium flame. Then, add the chopped onions. In about five minutes, they will soften and appear to be translucent. Then, add the red pepper, carrots, sugar, and sea salt to the skillet and keep cooking. Stir the mixture from time to time. In fifteen minutes, everything will be well caramelized. Then, add the tomato paste and the garlic and let the mixture cook for three minutes or until you get a caramelized fragrance from the paste.
2. Then, add the lentils, miso, and water to the skillet and bring the mixture to a boil. Once the mixture is boiling, reduce the flame and keep the skillet uncovered while the lentils are cooking. This will take about twenty-five to thirty minutes. Keep stirring the lentils from time to time, and in case they look dry, add some water. After that, add the cherry tomatoes and keep stirring.

3. While you are cooking the lentils, take a large pot and fill it with water. Add generous amounts of salt and bring the water to a boil. Then, add the chickpea pasta into the water and cook it for about five to six minutes or until al dente. Don't overcook it. Once done, drain the water and set them aside to cool.
4. Divide the penne into four to six meal prep containers and top with Bolognese. Sprinkle a few sage leaves or a bit of parmesan if you want.

Kale, Lemon, and White Bean Soup

Total Prep & Cooking Time: 1 hour 30 minutes

Yields: 2 servings

Nutrition Facts: Calories: 574 | Protein: 22g | Fat: 16g | Carbs: 106g | Fiber: 23g

Ingredients:

One hundred fifty grams of dried cannellini beans

Two cups of vegetable stock

Five cups of water

One white onion (large-sized, diced)

Two tbsps. of olive oil

Eight cloves of garlic

Kombu (one-inch strip)

One tsp. of dried thyme

Two potatoes (small ones, cubed after peeling)

Two bay leaves

One cup of kale

One lemon (juiced and zest)

Method:

1. Take an ample amount of water to soak the dried beans and keep them soaked for about twelve hours. Drain the beans properly and they should become double their size. Rinse them and they are ready to be cooked.
2. Take a large-sized pot, and in it, add one tbsp. of oil and heat it. Then, add the diced onion in the pot and cook the onions until they become golden and soft.
3. Then, add the stock and water along with garlic, dried beans, kombu, thyme, and bay leaves. Keep the pot covered and then bring it to a boil. Once it starts boiling, reduce the flame to a simmer and wait for about forty minutes.
4. While it is cooking, start with the kale. Wash it thoroughly. All the inner stalks that are tough should be removed. Then, start slicing them into ribbons of one-inch each. It looks good when you have delicate small pieces, so you should take your time with this.
5. After about half an hour, add the potatoes to the pot and then let the preparation simmer for ten more minutes. After this, both the potatoes and the beans should be soft. Take out the kombu and bay leaves.

Take a potato masher and use it carefully to mash at least half of the beans and potatoes.
6. Add the kale. Cook the mixture for ten more minutes. The water content needs to be checked now and see whether it is right or whether it needs to be topped up a bit. If the water is too much, then cook uncovered for a few minutes so that it dries up.
7. Once you notice the kale softening, take a tbsp. of olive oil and add it to the pot. Stir in the zest and lemon juice as well, and your dish is ready.

Broccoli Quinoa Casserole

Total Prep & Cooking Time: 45 minutes

Yields: 5 servings

Nutrition Facts: Calories: 491 | Protein: 27.6g | Fat: 16g | Carbs: 61.3g | Fiber: 9g

Ingredients:

Four and a half cups of vegetable stock

Two and a half cups of quinoa (uncooked)

Half a tsp. of salt

Two tablespoons of pesto sauce

Two teaspoons of cornstarch

Twelve ounces of mozzarella cheese (skimmed)

Two cups of spinach (fresh and organic)

One-third cup of parmesan cheese

Three medium-sized green onions (chopped)

Twelve ounces of broccoli florets (fresh)

Method:

1. Set the temperature of the oven to 400 degrees Fahrenheit and preheat. Take a rectangular baking dish and add the quinoa to it along with the green onions. In the meantime, take a large-sized bowl and add the broccoli florets to it. Microwave the florets at high for about five minutes. Once done, set them aside.
2. Take a large-sized mixing bowl and in it, add the pesto, vegetable sauce, cornstarch, and salt. Use a wire whisk to mix all of them properly. Now, heat this mixture until it starts to boil. You can either do this in the microwave, or you can use your stovetop as well.
3. Now, take the vegetable stock and the spinach and add them to the quinoa. Add the three-quarter of the mozzarella cheese and the parmesan as well. Bake the mixture for thirty to thirty-five minutes. Once done, take the casserole of quinoa out and then mix the broccoli into it. Take the rest of the cheese and sprinkle on top. Place the preparation back in the oven for another five minutes. By this time, all the cheese will melt.

Fish and Seafood

Fish and different types of seafood have a lot of essential nutrients in them and, thus, must be a part of your meal prepping. They also help in boosting brain health and they also have high levels of Vitamin D. They also contain omega-3-fatty acids which are beneficial to heart health.

Shrimp Fajita

Total Prep & Cooking Time: 20 minutes

Yields: 5 servings

Nutrition Facts: Calories: 203 | Protein: 16g | Fat: 8g | Carbs: 18g | Fiber: 7g

Ingredients:

For the fajita seasoning,

Half a tsp. of cayenne pepper

Half a tbsp. of chili powder

One tsp. each of

- Cumin powder
- Paprika

- Black pepper (freshly ground)
- Salt

For the shrimp,

One lb. of shrimp (shelled and deveined)

One tsp. of garlic

Two tbsps. of olive oil

Two pieces each of

- Yellow bell peppers (finely sliced)
- Red bell peppers (finely sliced)
- Green bell peppers (finely sliced)

One onion (medium-sized, chopped)

Cauliflower rice

To taste – black pepper and salt

Method:

1. Take all the ingredients of the fajita seasoning in one place and mix them together in a small bowl. Once done, set the bowl aside.
2. Take another large-sized bowl, and in it, add half of the fajita seasoning that you made along with the shrimp.

Mix and toss well and set it aside for about fifteen minutes.

3. Take a skillet of large size and pour olive oil in it. Place the skillet on high flame. Add the garlic, too and then cook it for about thirty seconds. After that, add the shrimp and keep stirring for five minutes. By the end of the time, the shrimp should be properly cooked. Once done, set it aside too.
4. Add some more olive oil in that same skillet and add the bell peppers, onions, and the remaining of the fajita seasoning that you have.
5. Stir fry the mixture for about five to ten minutes and do this on high heat.
6. Then, take four to five meal prep containers and divide everything equally, starting with the cauliflower rice and then the shrimp. Divide the veggies too.

Salmon Cobb Salad

Total Prep & Cooking Time: 45 minutes

Yields: 4 servings

Nutrition Facts: Calories: 427 | Protein: 24.8g | Fat: 29.6g | Carbs: 12g | Fiber: 5g

Ingredients:

Eight bacon slices

Four eggs (large-sized)

Two-three fillets of salmon (each of four oz. approx.)

One avocado (a large one, sliced)

Eight cups of romaine lettuce

Four tablespoons of red wine vinegar

Two tablespoons of olive oil

One pint of halved grape tomatoes

To taste – pepper and salt

Method:

1. Set the temperature of the oven to 350 degrees Fahrenheit and preheat. Take aluminum foil and use it to line your baking sheet. Now, take the salmon fillets and place them on the baking sheet. Season with black pepper and salt. Bake the preparation for about fifteen minutes, after which it will become tender and bright pink. Use a fork to flake the fish and set it aside.
2. Now, boil the eggs for ten minutes. Peel them after rinsing in cold water. Cut them in quarter shaped pieces and then keep them aside.
3. Take a non-stick skillet to prepare the bacon. Cook it for seven to eight minutes in the skillet over high heat. Flip the pieces once halfway through the process until they have become crispy and brown. Then, take a paper towel and transfer the bacon onto them to drain properly. After that, make large chunks by crumbling the bacon.
4. Take all the remaining vegetables and chop them after washing.
5. Then, it is time to make the red wine vinaigrette by adding one tablespoon of olive oil to one tablespoon of red wine vinegar. Mix them well and set them aside.
6. Now, it is time to prepare the containers. Start by dividing the lettuce first. Then, add the avocado, tomatoes, bacon bits, salmon, and eggs. Keep the dressing in a separate container at the side. If needed, sprinkle a bit of pepper and salt on top.

Asparagus Shrimp Stir Fry

Total Prep & Cooking Time: 50 minutes

Yields: 4 servings

Nutrition Facts: Calories: 236 | Protein: 23g | Fat: 4.5g | Carbs: 22g | Fiber: 3g

Ingredients:

One tbsp. of olive oil

One cup of brown rice

One lb. of asparagus (cut into one-inch pieces after trimming)

One and a half lbs. of shrimp (medium-sized)

One green onion (finely sliced)

One tsp. of sesame seeds

For the sauce,

Two tbsps. of oyster sauce

Three tbsps. of soy sauce (reduced-sodium variety)

One tbsp. each of

- Ginger (freshly grated)
- Brown sugar
- Rice wine vinegar

Three minced cloves of garlic

One tsp. each of

- Cornstarch
- Sesame oil

Method:

1. Take a small-sized bowl and in it, add the soy sauce, brown sugar, rice wine vinegar, oyster sauce, sesame oil, garlic, ginger, and cornstarch. Whisk all of these properly and set the bowl aside.
2. Take a saucepan of large size and then add two cups of water in it. Follow the instructions mentioned in the package and cook the rice accordingly. Set the rice aside.
3. Take a large-sized skillet and heat olive oil in it. Then, add the shrimp and keep stirring. Cook the shrimp for around three minutes. Then, add the asparagus pieces and keep stirring for another three minutes until all of it becomes tender.

4. Then, add the mixture of soy sauce and keep stirring to combine well. After one to two minutes, the sauce will thicken slightly.
5. Place the rice in the meal prep containers and the shrimp in another compartment of the same containers. Sprinkle green onions and sesame seeds on top for garnishing, but this is optional.

Shrimp Boil Skillet

Total Prep & Cooking Time: 35 minutes

Yields: 4 servings

Nutrition Facts: Calories: 393 | Protein: 31g | Fat: 18g | Carbs: 28g | Fiber: 4g

Ingredients:

Two tablespoons each of

- Olive oil
- Butter (made into small cubes)

One pound of yellow potatoes (baby ones)

Six ounces of sliced chicken smoked sausage

Half a yellow onion (large-sized, nicely chopped)

Two minced cloves of garlic

Three-quarter pounds of shrimp (peeled and deveined)

Two teaspoons of seafood seasoning

One and a quarter cups of fresh corn

Half a teaspoon of dried thyme

One tablespoon each of

- Fresh parsley (nicely minced)
- Lemon juice (freshly made)

Optional – Four ounces of fresh spinach

To taste – Pepper and salt

Method:

1. Take a large plate and place the potatoes on it. Microwave them for two minutes on high power.
2. Take them out, turn them, and microwave again for two minutes or even more until they become tender. Once done, let them cool a bit before making slices.
3. At the same time, take a large-sized non-stick skillet and heat olive oil in it. Add the chopped onions and then sauté them for four minutes. Take a spatula and push the chopped onions to the sides of the pan, and in the center, add the potatoes.
4. Use pepper and salt to season and keep turning the ingredients while cooking. After a while, they will turn golden brown. This will take about three minutes. Once done, push the potatoes to the side of the onions too.
5. Then, to the other side, add the sausages and keep tossing while cooking them. In about three minutes,

they will start to brown. Add the garlic and sauté for a minute more.

6. Now, add corn, shrimp, and butter to the skillet. Sprinkle the thyme and seafood seasoning as well. Add pepper and salt based on taste.
7. Keep tossing and cook for another two minutes. After that, add the spinach and keep stirring for two minutes, after which the spinach will start wilting. At this point, the shrimp should also have been cooked through.
8. Add some lemon juice and then toss them. If you want, garnish with some parsley.

Tuna Salad

Total Prep & Cooking Time: 20 minutes

Yields: 4 servings

Nutrition Facts: Calories: 227 | Protein: 13g | Fat: 11g | Carbs: 16g | Fiber: 3g

Ingredients:

Half a cup of Greek yogurt (non-fat variety)

A quarter cup each of

- Diced red onion
- Diced celery

Two tuna cans (each of five oz. drained and flaked)

One tbsp. each of

- Sweet pickle relish
- Dijon mustard

One sliced cucumber

One tsp. of lemon juice (freshly made)

Two eggs (large-sized)

A quarter tsp. of garlic powder

Four lettuce leaves

One sliced apple

Half a cup of raw almonds

To taste – Pepper (freshly ground) and salt

Method:

1. Take a medium-sized bowl and in it, add the celery, Greek yogurt, onion, garlic powder, lemon juice, relish pickle, and Dijon mustard. Mix them well and season with pepper and salt.
2. Then, take a large-sized saucepan and place your eggs in it. Then, pour one inch of cold water. Bring the water to a boil and cook the egg for a minute. Then, put a lid that tightly sits on the pan and set the pan aside for around ten minutes. After that, drain the excess water, peel the eggs, halve them, and set them aside.
3. Take the meal prep containers and place the lettuce leaves first followed by the mixture of tuna and then eggs, cucumber, almond, and apple.

Shrimp Stir Fry

Total Prep & Cooking Time: 30 minutes

Yields: 4 servings

Nutrition Facts: Calories: 276 | Protein: 24g | Fat: 7g | Carbs: 30g | Fiber: 7g

Ingredients:

Four cups of mixed vegetables (you can use broccoli and pepper)

Four tbsps. of vegetable oil

Two minced cloves of garlic

Three-quarter lbs. of shrimp (deveined and peeled)

Half a teaspoon of ginger (freshly grated)

Sesame seeds or green onions for garnishing

For the sauce,

One tbsp. of soy sauce

One tsp. of sesame oil

Half a cup of chicken broth

One tbsp. of cornstarch

Two tbsps. of hoisin sauce

Method:

1. First, take all the ingredients of the sauce in one place and then whisk them together so that they are mixed properly. Once done, set the sauce aside.
2. Take a frying pan and place it over medium flame. Heat two tsps. of oil in it. Add pepper, salt, and the shrimp and cook the shrimp well until it turns pink. This will take about two to three minutes. Once done, take the shrimp off the pan and keep it aside.
3. Take the remaining oil and heat it on high flame. Add all the vegetables and keep cooking until they turn crisp. This will take around four minutes. After that, add the ginger and garlic and keep stirring for another thirty seconds more.
4. Then, stir in the shrimp in the veggies and add the sauce too. Cook for about two minutes and keep stirring constantly. After that, you will see that the sauce is thickening.
5. Then, divide it after it has cooled down into the meal prep containers.

Healthy Snacks and Desserts

Snacks are what you need when you are always on the go, and everyone loves some dessert after a meal. But are these things healthy? Well, they can be if you use the right ingredients for them.

Frozen Banana Bites

Total Prep & Cooking Time: 2 hours 15 minutes

Yields: 48 bites

Nutrition Facts: Calories: 76 | Protein: 1.8g | Fat: 5.1g | Carbs: 6.9g | Fiber: 1g

Ingredients:

A cup of peanut butter

One-third cup of toffee baking bits

One oz. of semisweet chocolate

Four bananas (cut into rounds of one-inch thickness)

One tbsp. of shortening

Method:

1. First, take a wax paper and cover the baking sheet.
2. Then, take each slice of banana and layer with one spoon of peanut butter. Take a toothpick and insert it through the banana piercing through the layer of peanut butter. Then, take the banana bites and arrange them nicely on the baking sheet. Freeze the preparation for at least thirty minutes or overnight.
3. Now, melt the chocolate and keep stirring it frequently. To avoid any form of scorching, use a spatula to scrape down the sides continuously.
4. Take another waxed paper to cover another baking sheet.
5. Take two to four bites of bananas from the freezer at a time and then use the chocolate mixture to coat them. Now, take the coated bites and place them on this baking sheet that you just covered with wax paper. On top of each coated banana, sprinkle some toffee bits. Do the same process with all the bites. Now, return the preparation into the freezer and keep it there for at least an hour. Before serving, keep the bites at room temperature for around ten to fifteen minutes.

Italian Kale Chips

Total Prep & Cooking Time: 15 minutes

Yields: 2 servings

Nutrition Facts: Calories: 148 | Protein: 6g | Fat: 9g | Carbs: 15g | Fiber: 5g

Ingredients:

Four cups of kale (stems removed, loosely torn)

One-eighth tsp. each of

- Salt
- Pepper
- Garlic powder

A quarter tsp. of Italian seasoning

One tbsp. of olive oil

Optional – One tbsp. of grated Parmesan cheese

Method:

1. Set the temperature of the oven to 225 degrees Fahrenheit and preheat. The temperature of the oven is very important in this recipe; otherwise, your kale chips might just get burnt.
2. Now, it is time to prepare the kale. Tear the leaves and remove the stems. The leaves should be torn into bite-sized pieces.
3. Then, take a baking sheet and use cooking spray to coat it. After that, take the kale leaves and arrange them on the sheet in a single layer. Drizzle some more oil. Remember that too much oil can make the kale chips soggy, so be aware of how much oil you are using.
4. Now, take a small-sized bowl and in it, add garlic powder, Italian seasoning, pepper, and salt and mix them together. After mixing thoroughly, sprinkle this mixture evenly over the kale.
5. Once all of this is done, take the kale preparation and bake it for twelve minutes. After that, take them out, toss them a bit so that they get turned, and then return the preparation to the oven again. Bake for another five to ten minutes. By this time, the kale should be crispy. But keep a close eye on them since you don't want the burnt.
6. Once done, remove, and if you want, then sprinkle some grated Parmesan on top.

Apple and Quinoa Bars

Total Prep & Cooking Time: 1 hour

Yields: 12 servings

Nutrition Facts: Calories: 230 | Protein: 7g | Fat: 10g | Carbs: 31g | Fiber: 4g

Ingredients:

A quarter cup of peanut butter

One cup each of

- Apple sauce (unsweetened)
- Coconut oil

One tsp. of vanilla

Half a tsp. each of

- Baking powder
- Cinnamon

Two eggs

One and a half cups each of

- Rolled oats
- Quinoa (cooked and cooled)

One apple (chopped after peeling)

Method:

1. Set the temperature of the oven to 350 degrees Fahrenheit and preheat.
2. Take a baking dish of 8 by 8 inches and coat it with oil. After that, keep it aside.
3. Take a large-sized bowl and add the peanut butter, apple sauce, eggs, coconut oil, cinnamon, and vanilla in it and mix them all together.
4. Now, take the cooked quinoa and mix it too along with the baking powder and rolled oats. Keep mixing until everything is properly incorporated.
5. Then, fold the apple in.
6. After that, scoop out the mixture and spread it on the prepared baking dish. Make sure that it has covered every corner evenly.
7. Bake the preparation for about forty minutes. After it is done, a toothpick inserted should come out without anything on it.
8. Before you slice or store it, the bars should have cooled completely.

Note: You can store the preparation in the refrigerator for almost six days, and if you freeze it, they will stay fresh for three months.

Avocado Toast

Total Prep & Cooking Time: 5 minutes

Yields: 4 servings

Nutrition Facts: Calories: 156.4 | Protein: 5.1g | Fat: 8g | Carbs: 13.3g | Fiber: 4g

Ingredients:

One garlic clove

Four slices of bread (whole wheat variety)

One tsp. of parsley (finely chopped)

Juice of half a lemon

One avocado

To taste – Pepper and salt

For toppings – One tsp. of hemp seeds and some olive oil

Method:

1. Start by toasting the sliced of bread and use a toaster to do so. You can also do it on the stove. Once you have toasted them based on your preference, remove and place them on the plates.
2. Take the avocado and slice it in half. First, remove the pit and then use a spoon to scoop out the flesh of the avocado. Take a small bowl and put the flesh in it. Then, season with pepper and salt and add the juice of half a lemon. Then, add the parsley.
3. Use a fork to make a creamy mash of the avocado mixture and make sure that all the ingredients have combined well.
4. Take the garlic clove and crush it with the help of a fork. Remove the peel and then take the inside of the garlic and rub it a bit on top of the toasts.
5. Then, scoop out the avocado mash you made and spread them evenly on the slices. If you want, you can sprinkle some hemp seeds on top and drizzle a bit of olive oil.

Tuna Protein Box

Total Prep & Cooking Time: 20 minutes

Yields: 4 servings

Nutrition Facts: Calories: 414 | Protein: 27g | Fat: 25g | Carbs: 20g | Fiber: 3g

Ingredients:

Four carrots (chopped and peeled)

Four whole eggs

One cup of grapes

Two to three celery ribs (chopped nicely)

One cup of blueberries

Eight ounces of cubed cheese

For the tuna salad,

Two tbsps. each of

- Finely chopped celery
- Mayonnaise

Five ounces of drained tuna

Pepper and salt to taste

Method:

1. Firstly, cook the eggs and make them hard-boiled. Leave them to cool and then peel them.
2. Take all the ingredients of the tuna salad and stir them all together. Once done, divide the preparation among all the four meal prep containers.
3. Take all the other ingredients as well and divide them among the containers.
4. You can refrigerate the meal for up to four days if you refrigerate.

Note: You can enjoy this cold.

Puffed Quinoa Bars

Total Prep & Cooking Time: 40 minutes

Yields: 16 servings

Nutrition Facts: Calories: 98 | Protein: 3g | Fat: 4g | Carbs: 13g | Fiber: 2g

Ingredients:

Three cups of quinoa (puffed)

Half a cup each of

- Nut butter
- Packed soft dates
- Non-dairy milk

A quarter cup of cacao powder

Half a tsp. each of

- Sea salt
- Cinnamon

Method:

1. Take a square baking pan of 8 inches and then use parchment paper to line it properly. Take a large-sized mixing bowl and place the quinoa in it.
2. Put the nut butter and dates in a food processor and blend on high. Blend it so that the mixture becomes completely smooth. Then, add cacao, milk, salt, and cinnamon. Pulse again until everything has blended properly.
3. Then, add this mixture of dates into the quinoa puffs and keep mixing to ensure everything has combined well. Then, take this mixture and press it into the baking pan that you lined. Press it so that it is as even as possible.
4. Now, take the baking pan and place it in the freezer for at least half an hour. Then take it out and refrigerate for two to three hours. After that, cut it into squares (approximately 16).

Note: Refrigerate them in an air-tight container.

Roasted Broccoli

Total Prep & Cooking Time: 30 minutes

Yields: 6 servings

Nutrition Facts: Calories: 211 | Protein: 9g | Fat: 12g | Carbs: 21g | Fiber: 7g

Ingredients:

Five tablespoons of olive oil or coconut oil

Three broccoli crowns (sliced into bite-sized florets)

Two tablespoons each of

- Grated parmesan
- Lemon juice (freshly made)

Four minced cloves of garlic

Pepper to taste

Method:

1. Set the temperature of the oven to 425 degrees Fahrenheit and preheat.
2. Prepare the florets of broccoli by slicing them into appropriate size and then place them all in a bowl.
3. Use coconut oil or olive oil to toss the broccoli florets along with pepper, salt, and garlic.
4. Now, arrange the broccoli evenly on a baking sheet.
5. Roast the preparation for about twenty to fifteen minutes.
6. Once done, remove the preparation from the oven and then sprinkle some parmesan cheese and lime juice on top.

Note: You can enjoy it as a side dish as well.

Tuna Patties

Total Prep & Cooking Time: 15 minutes

Yields: 2 servings

Nutrition Facts: Calories: 249 | Protein: 35g | Fat: 8g | Carbs: 8g | Fiber: 1g

Ingredients:

Ten oz. of tuna

One tbsp. of dried chives

One-third cup of panko or breadcrumbs

Half a tbsp. of dried dill

Two beaten eggs

One tbsp. of Dijon mustard

One tsp. of olive oil

To taste – Pepper and salt

Optional – lemon wedges

Method:

1. Start by draining the tuna.
2. Then, take a large bowl and in it, add all the ingredients to mix them together.
3. Then, take the mixture to form four patties with your palm. Start by rolling then into balls and then shape them into patties.
4. Take a non-stick pan and heat the oil over medium flame. Add the patties and sauté them.
5. Cook each side of the patties for at least three to four minutes until they turn crisp and golden brown in color.
6. Take the lemon wedges and drizzle some juice on top of the patties.

Note: If you want to go gluten-free, then substitute with gluten-free breadcrumbs.

Rosemary Keto Crackers

Total Prep & Cooking Time: 50 minutes

Yields: 20 servings (5 crackers each serving)

Nutrition Facts: Calories: 111 | Protein: 5.9g | Fat: 9.2g | Carbs: 1.2g | Fiber: 1g

Ingredients:

6.2 ounces of almond flour

Four tablespoons of hemp seeds

One and two-thirds cup of parmesan cheese

Half a teaspoon of onion powder

Two tablespoons of rosemary (chopped)

One ounce of butter

Two large-sized eggs

Half a teaspoon of salt

Method:

1. Set the temperature of the oven to 375 degrees Fahrenheit and preheat.
2. In a mixing bowl, add all the dried ingredients. Whisk gently, but make sure that there are no lumps remaining.
3. Now, take a jug that is microwave-safe and place the butter in it. Melt the butter in the microwave. Add the eggs in this jug. Whisk the mixture until it becomes smooth.
4. Add this egg mixture onto the dry ingredients and mix thoroughly. A dough will form. At first, the dough can seem crumbly but keep pressing. Don't add any sort of liquids to the dough.
5. Keep the size of your over trays in mind and tear the baking paper accordingly. Now, take the dough and divide it in half. In case you are using smaller trays, divide it into quarters. Form the dough in the shape of a ball and place it on the baking paper.
6. Take another sheet and cover the dough. Use your rolling pin to press the dough. The layer should be around 3 millimeters. Once you have rolled them evenly, use a knife to form the shapes.
7. Cook them in the oven for about fifteen minutes.

Chapter 5:
30-Day Meal Prep Plan for Weight Loss

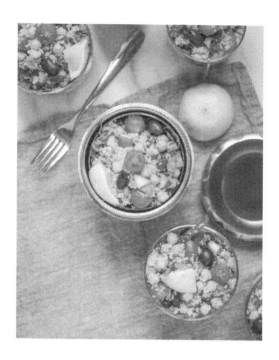

It is very easy to lose weight with meal prepping because counting calories becomes so much easier and you can exercise full portion control so that you don't end up adding up any hidden calories than planned. And if you think that it is going to take up a lot of time from your schedule, then you are wrong because, with this 30-day meal plan, meal prepping will become so much easier. Once you get the hang of it, you can also try out new recipes from the ones mentioned in the previous chapters.

Week 1

Breakfast – Low Carb Waffles

Total Prep & Cooking Time: 10 minutes

Yields: 4 servings

Nutrition Facts: Calories: 264 | Protein: 14g | Fat: 22g | Carbs: 6g | Fiber: 3g

Ingredients:

Two mashed bananas

Six eggs (large-sized)

Three tablespoons of quinoa or rice flour

Cooking spray

Two tablespoons of almond butter (unsweetened)

Half a teaspoon of ground cinnamon

For toppings,

Half a tablespoon each of

- Almond butter
- Coconut butter
- Chopped walnuts

A quarter of a banana (cut into slices)

One tablespoon of maple syrup or honey

Method:

1. Firstly, heat the waffle iron. Then, take a large-sized bowl and in it, add the almond butter, mashed bananas, eggs, flour, and cinnamon and mix them well by whisking. Whisk until everything is smooth. Season with salt.
2. Then, use cooking spray to grease the waffle iron and add one-third cup of batter. Cook until the waffle is golden. Repeat with the rest of the batter.
3. Keep the remaining waffles in the fridge in air-tight containers. Use toppings of your choice.

Lunch – Avocado Basil Shrimp Wraps

Total Prep & Cooking Time: 50 minutes

Yields: 4 servings

Nutrition Facts: Calories: 202 | Protein: 12g | Fat: 14g | Carbs: 7g | Fiber: 2g

Ingredients:

For the sweet potato chips,

Two to three sweet potatoes (medium-sized, sliced into coins)

Cooking spray

Kosher salt to taste

A pinch of black pepper (freshly ground)

For the shrimp,

Twenty shrimps (large-sized, deveined, peeled)

A quarter of red onion (small-sized, diced finely)

One and a half cups of halved grape tomatoes

Two avocados (finely diced)

Two romaine lettuce heads

Four leaves of basil (fresh, sliced thinly)

Cooking spray

For the marinade,

Two minced cloves of garlic

Three tablespoons of olive oil (extra-virgin variety)

Three leaves of basil (sliced thinly)

Two tablespoons of white wine vinegar

Two lemons (juiced)

Half a teaspoon of paprika

Kosher salt to taste

A pinch of black pepper (freshly ground)

Method:

1. First, start by making the sweet potato chips. Set the temperature of the oven to 375 degrees Fahrenheit and then take a large baking sheet. Grease it with the help

of cooking spray. Now, arrange the slices of sweet potatoes evenly on it and season with pepper and salt.

2. Roast the potatoes for fifteen minutes. Take them out, flip them, and then roast them for another fifteen minutes. Once done, let them cool and then put them in one of the compartments of the meal prep containers.

3. Now, make the shrimp salad. Take a large skillet and place it on medium flame. Drizzle with cooking spray. Add the shrimp and keep stirring. Cook it for two minutes and make sure that it is no longer opaque. Once done, set the shrimp aside and let it cool.

4. Then, make the marinade. Take a small-sized bowl and in it, add the garlic, lemon juice, basil, oil, vinegar, paprika, pepper, and salt and whisk everything together.

5. Take another large-sized bowl and in it, add the avocados, onions, tomatoes, and basil. Add the shrimp. Mix them well. Then, drizzle the marinade on top. Toss everything to coat them properly with the marinade.

6. Now divide the shrimp salad evenly among the four meal prep containers and place them in lettuce cups.

Snacks – Peanut Butter Granola Bars

Total Prep & Cooking Time: 22 minutes

Yields: 12 servings

Nutrition Facts: Calories: 204 | Protein: 4g | Fat: 11g | Carbs: 21g | Fiber: 2g

Ingredients:

A quarter cup each of

- Peanut butter (all-natural)
- Mini chocolate chips (keep some more for toppings)

One-third cup of honey

A quarter cup of coconut oil

A pinch of salt

One tsp. of vanilla extract

Two cups of rolled oats

Half a cup of almonds

Method:

1. Take a baking sheet of 8 by 8 inches and use parchment paper to line it. Use some cooking spray and then set the pan aside.
2. Take a saucepan of medium size and in it, add peanut butter, honey, and coconut oil. Combine the ingredients well by heating on medium flame. Keep stirring until the mixture is smooth.
3. After that, bring the flame to a simmer and cook for another one minute by stirring frequently. Then, remove the pan from the flame and stir in the salt and vanilla. After mixing, allow the mixture to cool down for ten to fifteen minutes.
4. Once the mixture has cooled a bit, add the rolled oats, almonds, and chocolate chips. Stir properly.
5. Now, take this mixture and spread it properly on the baking sheet. Use a spatula to press and spread it. You can use a bit of oil on the spatula so that the mixture does not stick to it while pressing.
6. Take a few more mini chocolate chips and sprinkle them on top. After that, refrigerate the mixture for at least a period of two hours. Once the time is over, take them out and cut into bars.

Note: You can refrigerate the bars for at least two weeks if stored in air-tight containers. These are not only crunchy but also flavorful, and you don't have to bake them as well.

Dinner – Beef and Broccoli

The recipe for this has already been mentioned in the previous chapter here.

If you have a craving for takeout, then this beef and broccoli is definitely going to satisfy your cravings and it is a much healthier option too. You can also tweak this recipe by adding your favorite veggies like carrots or bell pepper or even mushrooms if you want.

Week 2

Breakfast – Avocado Quinoa Frittatas

The recipe has been mentioned in the previous chapter here.

If you want, you can throw in a bit of sausage in these frittatas as well, and they taste heavenly with a bit of hot sauce.

Lunch – Collard Wrap Bento Boxes

Total Prep & Cooking Time: 20 minutes

Yields: 4 servings

Nutrition Facts: Calories: 348 | Protein: 10g | Fat: 15g | Carbs: 32g | Fiber: 12g

Ingredients:

Four tablespoons of hummus

Two carrots (medium-sized, sliced into matchsticks after peeling)

One cucumber (medium-sized, cut after peeling)

Two avocados (sliced after removing the pit)

One cup of purple cabbage (shredded)

Three ounces of sautéed tofu or shredded chicken

Four collard leaves (large-sized, ribs have to be removed)

For each bento box,

Half a cup of berries or grapes

One cup of mixed celery sticks and carrots

One ounce of 70% dark chocolate

Method:

1. Take one collard leaf, and in the middle of it, spread one tbsp. of the hummus. Now, divide the tofu or chicken and the veggies equally among the collard leaves. Then, gently roll the leaves and form a neat wrap.
2. Cut each wrap in half and place them in one of the compartments of the bento box.

Snacks – Chocolate Barks

Total Prep & Cooking Time: 1 hour 15 minutes

Yields: 24 servings

Nutrition Facts: Calories: 100 | Protein: 1.7g | Fat: 7.5g | Carbs: 9.2g | Fiber: 1.3g

Ingredients:

Twelve ounces of dark chocolate chips

A quarter cup each of

- Unsalted pistachios (chopped roughly)
- Coconut flakes (unsweetened)
- Dried cherries

Half a cup of chopped salted pretzels

Flaky sea salt

Method:

1. Take a parchment paper and line your baking sheet. Then, melt the dark chocolate chips and pour one-third

of it in the baking sheet. Spread into an even layer with the help of a spatula.
2. Sprinkle the cherries, pretzels, pistachios, and coconut on top evenly.
3. Take the remaining dark chocolate and pour it on top of these ingredients. Make sure it forms an even layer.
4. Sprinkle the remaining ingredients on top. Lastly, use sea salt for garnishing.
5. Let this bark cool, and for that, keep it like that for an hour. After that, break it into pieces. Store the barks in the air-tight containers.

Dinner – Zoodle Ramen

Total Prep & Cooking Time: 20 minutes

Yields: 4 servings

Nutrition Facts: Calories: 195 | Protein: 9.6g | Fat: 12.3g | Carbs: 12.1g | Fiber: 3g

Ingredients:

One tablespoon each of

- Olive oil (extra virgin variety)
- Soy sauce (low-sodium variety)
- Sesame oil

Eight ounces of cremini mushrooms (thinly sliced)

Eight cups of bone broth (low-sodium variety)

Half a cup of red cabbage (chopped)

Four zucchinis (medium-sized, spiralized to form noodles)

Four minced cloves of garlic

One teaspoon of freshly minced ginger

Two thinly sliced green onions

Two tablespoons of sesame seeds (toasted)

One cup of carrots (shredded)

Four eggs (large-sized)

Red pepper flakes

Method:

1. Take a small pot and place the eggs in it. Pour cold water so that they cover the eggs by an inch. Now, plate the pot on your stovetop and bring the water to a boil. Once it starts boiling, turn the flame off and keep the pot covered. Let it stay like that for eleven minutes.
2. After that, take the eggs out of the pot and dip them in cold water. After peeling, cut them in half lengthwise.
3. Place a large skillet on medium flame and add the olive oil it. Heat the oil. Then, add the mushrooms and keep stirring. Cook them for about five minutes. By this time, the mushrooms will become soft. Add the ginger and garlic and cook them for another minute.
4. Then, take the bone broth and add it to the skillet. Add the soy sauce too, and then bring the mixture to a boil. Once it starts boiling, reduce the flame to a simmer and let it stay like that for five minutes. After that, add the zucchini noodles. Keep cooking for two more minutes

until the zucchini noodles are tender. Then, add the sesame oil and keep stirring.
5. Now, take four mason jars or meal prep containers and divide the noodles and broth equally. Divide the hardboiled eggs, cabbage, and carrots as well.
6. Top each container with red pepper flakes, sesame seeds, and scallions.
7. Simply microwave before eating.

Week 3

Breakfast – Egg Muffins

Total Prep & Cooking Time: 55 minutes

Yields: 12 servings

Nutrition Facts: Calories: 173 | Protein: 10g | Fat: 13g | Carbs: 1g | Fiber: 1g

Ingredients:

Three slices of bacon (turkey)

Cooking spray

One red bell pepper (chopped)

One yellow onion (small-sized, chopped)

Six eggs (large-sized)

Two cups of baby spinach (finely chopped)

A quarter teaspoon of paprika

Half a teaspoon of garlic powder

Three tablespoons of milk

Half a cup of shredded mozzarella

To taste – black pepper (freshly ground) and salt

Method:

1. Set the temperature of the oven to 350 degrees Fahrenheit and preheat. Take a muffin tin of twelve cups and grease it with the help of cooking spray. Then, take a skillet (large-sized) and place it over medium flame. Cook the bacon in it for eight minutes until it turns crispy. Take a plate lined with a paper towel to drain the bacon. After that, crumble it.
2. Now, take the bell pepper and onion and add them to the skillet. Cook them for five minutes until they are soft. Then, add the spinach. Cook for two more minutes, and you will notice that the spinach starts to wilt.
3. Take a small-sized bowl and mix the following ingredients in it – milk, eggs, paprika, pepper, salt, and garlic powder. Whisk them together. Take the cooked vegetable mixture and add it to the eggs. Add the turkey bacon too. Mix them all well. Then add the mozzarella. Once you have combined everything, pour this mixture into the muffin tin.
4. Bake the mixture for about thirty to thirty-five minutes until it is completely cooked through.
5. Let the muffins cool before you store them in the containers.

Lunch – Steak Salad

Total Prep & Cooking Time: 30 minutes

Yields: 4 servings

Nutrition Facts: Calories: 321 | Protein: 18g | Fat: 25g | Carbs: 7g | Fiber: 3g

Ingredients:

Three-quarter tsps. of salt (keep it divided)

Half a tsp. of pepper (keep it divided)

Three-quarter lbs. of top sirloin steak or beef flat iron steak

A quarter cup of olive oil

Two tsps. of lemon juice

Two tbsps. of balsamic vinegar

One beefsteak tomato (medium-sized, sliced)

Five oz. of baby spinach (fresh, almost six cups)

Half an avocado (medium-sized, ripe, sliced after peeling)

Four radishes (sliced into thin strips)

Optional – A quarter cup of blue cheese (crumbled)

Method:

1. Firstly, sprinkle the steak with a quarter tsp. of pepper and half a tsp. of salt. Cover it and grill on medium heat. The meat should reach the desired state before you take it off. Let it stay aside for five minutes once done.
2. While you grill the steak, take a small-sized bowl and add vinegar, oil, lemon juice, and the remaining half of the pepper and salt. Whisk them all together.
3. Divide the spinach into the four meal prep containers. Add radishes, avocado, and tomato.
4. Once the steak is ready, cut it into slices and then place the slices over the salad after dividing it into four parts. Drizzle the dressing on top. And if you want, then use the blue cheese on top by sprinkling a bit.

Snacks – Mango Sorbet

Total Prep & Cooking Time: 3 hours 15 minutes

Yields: 4 servings

Nutrition Facts: Calories: 49 | Carbs: 12g | Fiber: 1g

Ingredients:

Three and a half cup of diced mangoes

A quarter cup of warm water

One teaspoon of lime juice (freshly squeezed)

Method:

1. Take a rimmed baking sheet and line the mangoes in it after dicing them neatly. The baking sheet must be covered with parchment paper.
2. Freeze the mangoes for three to four hours until they are completely frozen and solid. Or, you can keep them in the freezer overnight as well.
3. Now, take the frozen diced mangoes out and add them to a food processor. Add the lime juice as well.

4. Blend the mixture until it becomes smooth and creamy.
5. If needed, then you can add the warm water as it will help the process.
6. If you want a softer texture, then you can serve immediately or you can also store them in freezer-safe containers for later.

Dinner – Lentil Bolognese

The recipe is already mentioned in the previous chapter here.

Week 4

Breakfast – Strawberry Overnight Oats

Total Prep & Cooking Time: 2 hours 10 minutes

Yields: 4 servings

Nutrition Facts: Calories: 252 | Protein: 8g | Fat: 7g | Carbs: 39g | Fiber: 8g

Ingredients:

Two cups of almond milk

Two cups of rolled oats

A quarter cup of strawberry jam

One-third cup of peanut butter (unsweetened)

One tablespoon of honey

One cup of strawberries (chopped)

Method:

1. Take a large-sized mixing bowl and add the milk, oats, peanut butter, and honey to it and combine them well together. Cover the bowl and keep it in the refrigerator for at least two hours, or you can even keep them overnight.
2. Now, take the mixture and divide it equally among four jars.
3. Top the jars with a quarter cup of strawberries. Add two tbsps. of jam on top.

Lunch – One Pan Salmon and Asparagus

Total Prep & Cooking Time: 45 minutes

Yields: 4servings

Nutrition Facts: Calories: 319 | Protein: 9.6g | Fat: 4g | Carbs: 64.3g | Fiber: 9.9g

Ingredients:

Four salmon fillets

Three pounds of yellow potatoes

One bunch of asparagus

One teaspoon of garlic powder

One tablespoon of olive oil

Method:

1. Slice the potatoes into quarter shapes and arrange them on the baking sheet. Drizzle some olive oil and also sprinkle garlic powder on top. Bake the mixture at

420 degrees Fahrenheit in the oven for about twenty minutes.
2. Remove the preparation once done and then add the salmon and asparagus.
3. Bake the preparation again for about fifteen minutes, and your dish is ready.
4. Divide the potatoes, asparagus, and salmon equally into four air-tight meal prep containers.

Snacks – Pumpkin Pie Balls

Total Prep & Cooking Time: 45 minutes

Yields: 4servings

Nutrition Facts: Calories: 76 | Protein: 2g | Fat: 4g | Carbs: 9g | Fiber: 2g

Ingredients:

One cup of rolled oats

One-third cup of pumpkin puree (unsweetened)

Half a cup each of

- Almond butter (unsweetened, warmed)
- Coconut shavings or flakes

A quarter cup of golden raisins

Two tablespoons each of

- Pumpkin seeds
- Chia seeds
- Maple syrup

One teaspoon of pumpkin pie spice

Method:

1. Take a large-sized bowl and in it, add coconut, oats, pumpkin puree, almond butter, raisins, chia seeds, maple syrup, pumpkin pie spice, and pumpkin seeds and mix them together until everything has fully combined.
2. Now, use your hands to form balls from this mixture. Each ball should be around two inches. Once done, transfer the balls to a baking sheet.
3. Refrigerate these balls for half an hour until they are fully set.
4. Store them in air-tight meal prep containers.

Dinner – California Roll Sushi Bowls

Total Prep & Cooking Time: 40 minutes

Yields: 5 servings

Nutrition Facts: Calories: 465 | Protein: 10g | Fat: 8g | Carbs: 84g | Fiber: 6g

Ingredients:

Five tablespoons of rice vinegar (keep it divided)

Two cups of California sushi rice (dry)

Half a teaspoon of salt

One and a half tablespoon of sriracha

Two tablespoons of granulated sugar

A quarter cup each of

- Mayonnaise (light variety)
- Soy sauce (low-sodium variety)

Ten ounces of lump crabmeat (diced into small cubes)

Three-quarter cups of carrots (chopped into matchstick sizes)

One and a half tablespoons of sushi ginger (pickled)

One nori sheet (make small pieces by chopping)

One and a half cups of cucumber (chopped)

Sesame seeds (toasted, for garnishing)

One avocado (large-sized, diced)

Method:

1. Take a strainer with fine mesh and place the rice on it. Then, rinse it under cold water. Do it for about two minutes. After rinsing, take a medium-sized saucepan and transfer the rice to it and add two and a quarter cups of water to the saucepan. Place the pan on high heat and bring it to a boil. After that, cover the saucepan and reduce the flame to a simmer and let it be for fifteen minutes. After that, remove the saucepan from the flame and let it rest for another fifteen minutes. Don't uncover it before that.
2. Meanwhile, add four tablespoons of vinegar to a small-sized saucepan along with salt and sugar. Put it on medium flame and keep whisking until all the sugar has combined and dissolved fully. Then, remove the pan from the flame. Once the rice has fully cooled, add this mixture of vinegar over the rice. To coat it evenly, toss well.

3. Then, take a mixing bowl of small size and mix sriracha with mayonnaise in it by whisking. You can make the mixture thin by adding a tablespoon of water. Take a resealable bag of small size and transfer this mixture to it. Set it aside too.
4. Take another small-sized mixing bowl and add the remaining one tablespoon of vinegar in it along with soy sauce and then whisk the mixture. Once done, keep it aside. Take a large-sized mixing bowl and in it, add the crab meat, carrots, nori, cucumber, avocado, and ginger. Mix them well.
5. Then, take 4-5 meal prep containers and divide the rice. On top of the rice, add the crab mixture, followed by the mixture of soy sauce. Take the resealable bag and cut one small corner to pour the sriracha mixture.

Chapter 6:
Healthy Meals to Prep and Go

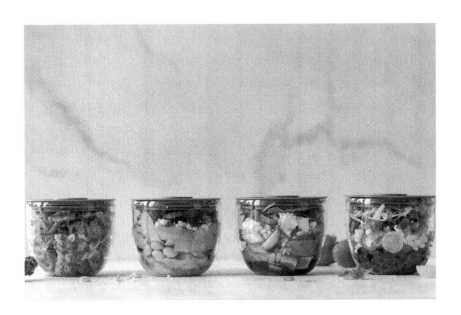

Weekdays can get really hectic, and you might not have time for elaborate meal prepping. That is why I have listed ten special recipes for you that you can easily prep and go.

Sheet Pan Cashew Chicken

Total Prep & Cooking Time: 30 minutes

Yields: 4 servings

Nutrition Facts: Calories: 251 | Protein: 12g | Fat: 11g | Carbs: 27g | Fiber: 2g

Ingredients:

For the sauce,

One tbsp. of hoisin sauce

Six tbsps. of soy sauce (low-sodium variety)

Two tbsps. each of

- Honey
- Arrowroot or cornstarch

Two minced cloves of garlic

Three-quarter tbsps. of apple cider vinegar

One tsp. of sesame oil (toasted)

Half a tsp. of ginger (freshly minced)

Half a cup of water

For the chicken,

One and a half cups of broccoli florets

Two chicken breasts or thighs (medium-sized, cut into cubes, skinless, boneless)

One red bell pepper

Two-thirds cup of cashews (roasted but unsalted)

To taste – black pepper and salt

Optional – half a green bell pepper

Method:

For the sauce,

Take a saucepan of medium size and in it, add the ingredients of the sauce and keep stirring. Once all of them have properly combined, bring the flame to a simmer. Keep stirring from time to time until the sauce gets thick. Once done, set aside to cool.

For the chicken and veggies,

1. Set the temperature of the oven to 400 degrees Fahrenheit and preheat. Use parchment paper to coat a large-sized baking sheet. Use cooking spray.
2. Take the chicken cubes and season with pepper and salt. Use spoonfuls of the sauce to drizzle on top of the chicken. Coat them well on all sides. Keep half of the sauce for use later on.
3. Cook the chicken in the preheated oven for eight minutes. After that, remove the pan.
4. Now, take the bell peppers, broccoli florets, and cashews and arrange them around the chicken in one

layer. Season with pepper and salt. Also, scoop the sauce and drizzle on top. Toss the chicken and veggies so that everything is well coated. Return the preparation to the oven and cook them for another ten to twelve minutes. By this time, the chicken should be fully cooked.

5. After you remove the chicken from the oven, drizzle any remaining sauce on top. Serve or store the chicken with quinoa. Sprinkle some sesame seeds and green onions on top if desired.

Almond Flour Pancakes

Total Prep & Cooking Time: 15 minutes

Yields: 12 servings

Nutrition Facts: Calories: 101 | Protein: 5.4g | Fat: 7.5g | Carbs: 2.8g | Fiber: 1.4g

Ingredients:

One cup of almond flour

Six eggs (keep them in room temperature)

A quarter cup each of

- Almond milk (unsweetened)
- Coconut flour

One teaspoon of baking powder

Half a teaspoon of vanilla extract

Method:

1. Place a skillet on medium flame and use non-stick cooking spray.
2. Take a mixing bowl and add the eggs to it along with vanilla and milk. Whisk them together.

3. Add coconut flour, almond flour, and baking powder. Mix properly until you get a smooth mixture. But make sure you don't overmix.
4. Take a quarter cup of the batter and pour it into the pan. Let it form the pancake. Repeat the same to form twelve pancakes.
5. Cook each side for two to three minutes, and then you need to flip them carefully and cook that side for another two to three minutes. The pancakes must achieve a golden brown color on both sides.
6. Once done, cool a bit before packing into containers.

Asian Lemon Chicken

Total Prep & Cooking Time: 30 minutes

Yields: 4 servings

Nutrition Facts: Calories: 320 | Protein: 26g | Fat: 4g | Carbs: 21g

Ingredients:

One pound of chicken breast (boneless, skinless, cubed)

One slightly beaten egg white

Three-fourth tsp. of salt

One-third cup of breadcrumbs

Half a cup of cornstarch flour

A quarter tsp. of black pepper

Oil

For the sauce,

A quarter cup of honey

One-third cup of soy sauce (low-sodium variety)

Three tbsps. each of

- Lemon juice (freshly made)
- Cornstarch
- Water

One tbsp. of lemon zest

Two tbsps. of rice wine vinegar

Two minced cloves of garlic

One tsp. of sesame oil

A quarter tsp. of ginger (freshly grated)

Half a tsp. of Sriracha hot sauce

For garnishing,

Sesame seeds

Finely chopped green onions

Method:

1. Take a medium-sized saucepan and mix all the ingredients of sauce in the pan. Take three tbsps. of the mixture and add to a large bowl. Keep the saucepan aside. Add the egg white to that same mixing bowl along with the cubes of chicken. Mix them well.

2. Take a zip-top bag of large size and add the breadcrumbs, cornstarch, black pepper, and salt to it. Add the chicken too. Lock the bag and shake it well.
3. Now, it is time to cook the chicken. Take two to three tbsps. of oil in a skillet and place it over medium-high flame. Add the chicken in batches and pan-fry them until they are golden brown in color. This will take about five minutes for each side. Then, take a large platter and line it with paper towels. Transfer the chicken onto the platter.
4. Now, while you are cooking the chicken, take a saucepan and add the sauce to it. Heat it, and when it starts bubbling, start whisking. When the sauce has thickened, turn the flame off. Season according to taste. If you want it tangier, then add some lemon. If you want it sweeter, then add honey. Or, you can add sriracha in case you want it spicier. Set it aside.
5. Once done, toss the chicken in the sauce that you had set aside. Ensure that they have coated well.
6. Garnish with sesame seeds and green onions and divide in meal prep containers along with some brown rice.

Berry Fruit Salad

Total Prep & Cooking Time: 10 minutes

Yields: 4 servings

Nutrition Facts: Calories: 181 | Protein: 3g | Fat: 1g | Carbs: 43g | Fiber: 11g

Ingredients:

Eight oz. each of

- Fresh blueberries
- Fresh blackberries

Two pints of halved strawberries

Four oz. of fresh raspberries

Two tbsps. of lime juice (fresh)

Half a cup of pomegranate seeds

One tbsp. of honey

A quarter tsp. of lime zest

Method:

1. Take a large-sized bowl and add the raspberries, blueberries, blackberries, and strawberries in it.
2. Take another separate bowl and in it, add the lime zest, lime juice, and honey and whisk them together.
3. Once the mixture is ready, pour it over the berries and toss everything gently so that they are all fully coated with this mixture.
4. You can chill it in the refrigerator for a couple of hours before serving, or you can even choose to have it immediately.

Deli Style Protein Box

Total Prep & Cooking Time: 10 minutes

Yields: 1 serving

Nutrition Facts: Calories: 382 | Protein: 23g | Fat: 25g | Carbs: 16g | Fiber: 3g

Ingredients:

Two oz. turkey breast slices

A quarter cup of cherry tomatoes

One hard-boiled egg (large-sized)

Four pita bites crackers

One oz. of shredded cheddar cheese

Two tbsps. of raw almonds

Method:

1. Place the tomatoes, turkey, crackers, egg, cheese, and almonds in the different compartments of the meal prep container.

Chicken Pesto Pasta

Total Prep & Cooking Time: 10 minutes

Yields: 1 serving

Nutrition Facts: Calories: 382 | Protein: 23g | Fat: 25g | Carbs: 16g | Fiber: 3g

Ingredients:

Three tbsps. of olive oil (keep it divided)

One lb. of trimmed asparagus

Half a cup each of

- Cherry tomatoes
- Basil pesto

One lb. each of

- Cubed chicken breasts (skinless, boneless)
- Penne pasta (whole-wheat variety)

Two tbsps. of parsley (freshly chopped)

To taste – black pepper (freshly ground) and kosher salt

Method:

1. Set the temperature of the oven to 425 degrees Fahrenheit and preheat. Take a baking sheet of large size and use oil to coat it.
2. Take the asparagus and arrange them nicely on the baking sheet and make sure that they are in a single layer.
3. Use two tbsps. of olive oil to drizzle on top. Season with pepper and salt. Toss the asparagus so that every piece is evenly combined with the seasonings. Place the baking sheet in the oven and roast the asparagus for about eight to twelve minutes. They should be crisp and yet tender when completed. Before slicing, let them cool.
4. Take a large pot and in it add water along with salt. Boil the water. Cook the pasta in the water and follow the instructions mentioned on its package. Once done, drain the pasta.
5. Put a large skillet on medium flame and heat the remaining one tbsp. of oil in it. Use pepper and salt to season the chicken. Then, add the chicken to the skillet and cook them for four minutes on each side until they golden brown in color. Set the chicken aside.
6. Take a large-sized bowl and in it, add the pasta, asparagus, pesto, tomatoes, and chicken. Combine well.
7. Once cooled, divide into meal prep containers and then use parsley for garnishing.

Simple Breakfast Meal Prep

Total Prep & Cooking Time: 50 minutes

Yields: 4 serving

Nutrition Facts: Calories: 360 | Protein: 21g | Fat: 24g | Carbs: 17g | Fiber: 3g

Ingredients:

Three tbsps. of olive oil (keep it divided)

Twelve oz. of russet potatoes (cubed)

Two minced cloves of garlic

Eight lightly beaten eggs

Half a tsp. of dried thyme

A quarter cup of Mexican blend cheese (shredded)

Twelve oz. of broccoli florets

Four bacon slices

To taste – pepper and salt

Method:

1. Set the temperature of the oven to 400 degrees Fahrenheit and preheat. Take a baking sheet and use oil to coat it lightly. You can also use non-stick cooking spray.
2. Now, take the cubes of potatoes and place them on the baking sheet and keep them in a single layer. Add one tbsp. of olive oil on top and sprinkle the thyme too. Add the garlic. Season with pepper and salt. Toss the potato cubes gently so that they become well combined.
3. Take the preparation and place it in the oven. Bake the potatoes for around thirty minutes. They must be crisp and golden brown. Once done, set them aside.
4. Take the remaining two tbsps. of oil and pour it over a large skillet. Place the skillet on medium flame and heat the oil. Add the eggs. Keep whisking them until they get set on the skillet. Season with pepper and salt. Keep cooking until you can no longer see any remains of the egg. This will take about five minutes. Use cheese for topping the egg.
5. Now, take the bacon and add it to the skillet. Cook the bacon until it is crispy and brown. This will take about eight minutes. Once done, line a plate with a paper towel and transfer the bacon onto it.
6. Take a pan of boiling water, and over it set a colander. Take the broccoli florets in it. Steam the broccoli in the

covered state for about five minutes until they appear vibrant green.
7. Now, arrange the bacon, eggs, potatoes, and broccoli into the various compartments of your meal prep containers.

Mason Jar Chicken Salad

Total Prep & Cooking Time: 15 minutes

Yields: 4 servings

Nutrition Facts: Calories: 283 | Protein: 26g | Fat: 10g | Carbs: 23g | Fiber: 4g

Ingredients:

For the salad,

Half a cup of toasted pecans

Eight chopped leaves of romaine lettuce

Two tsps. of freshly squeezed lemon juice

One apple (finely chopped)

Three chopped ribs of celery

One cup of halved grapes

Two chicken half breasts (skinless, boneless)

For the dressing,

One and a half tbsps. of apple cider vinegar

Three-quarter cups of Greek yogurt

One tbsp. each of

- Lemon juice
- Honey

One tsp. of poppy seeds

Two tbsps. of water

Pepper and salt to taste

Method:

1. First, cook the chicken. Take a large or medium-sized skillet and place it on medium flame. Use some cooking spray. Now, add the chicken. Season with pepper and salt. Cook each side of the chicken for at least two to three minutes until they are browned. Now, flip the chicken and cook the other side as well. After that, add some water so that the level of water is halfway up the chicken. Keep the skillet covered with the lid. Make sure the chicken is cooked fully.
2. Meanwhile, take all the dressing ingredients together and whisk them in a salad bowl. Taste the dressing and if needed, then add a bit more honey. Once done, divide the dressing among the four jars.
3. Take the apple pieces and toss them in lemon juice.

4. Once you, the prepared chicken has cooled down, cube them into small pieces.
5. Take the other salad ingredients and divide them equally among the four jars. Divide the chicken too. Seal the jars. Keep them in the refrigerator. Just before you eat the salad, shake it well and then pour it into a plate or a bowl.

Taco Meal Prep Bowl

Total Prep & Cooking Time: 60 minutes

Yields: 5 servings

Nutrition Facts: Calories: 255 | Protein: 40g | Fat: 28.4g | Carbs: 60g | Fiber: 9g

Ingredients:

Two tbsps. of olive oil

One cup of brown rice

Two packets of taco seasoning

Two lbs. of ground beef

Fifteen oz. of black beans (rinsed and drained)

One can of corn (15.25 oz.) (whole kernel, drained)

Three Roma tomatoes (roughly diced)

Method:

1. Take a saucepan of large size and add two cups of water to it. Follow the instructions mentioned on the package to cook the rice. Once done, set it aside.

2. Take a large stockpot and heat the oil in it on medium flame. Add the beef and cook it properly. It should turn brown within five minutes. As you are cooking the beef, make sure it crumbles. Add the taco seasoning. Remove all the excess fat.
3. Now, take the rice and divide it equally among the airtight meal prep containers. Place the beef mixture on top. Add the corn, black beans, and tomatoes.

Greek Chicken Meal Prep Bowls

Total Prep & Cooking Time: 1hour 30 minutes

Yields: 5 servings

Nutrition Facts: Calories: 481 | Protein: 42g | Fat: 30g | Carbs: 33g | Fiber: 3.3g

Ingredients:

One and a half lbs. of halved cherry tomatoes

One cup of brown rice

For the chicken,

A quarter cup of olive oil (keep two tbsps. extra)

Three minced cloves of garlic

Two lbs. of chicken breasts (skinless, boneless)

One lemon (juiced)

One tbsp. each of

- Dried oregano
- Red wine vinegar

To taste – black pepper and salt

For the tzatziki sauce,

One finely diced English cucumber

One tbsp. each of

- Lemon zest
- Fresh dill (chopped)

One tsp. each of

- Lemon zest
- Fresh mint (chopped)

Two tbsps. of olive oil

Two pressed cloves of garlic

One cup of Greek yogurt (plain)

To taste – pepper and salt

For the cucumber salad,

Two peeled and sliced English cucumbers

Two pressed cloves of garlic

Two tbsps. of olive oil

Half a cup of red onion (thinly sliced)

One lemon (juiced)

Half a tsp. of dried oregano

One tbsp. of red wine vinegar

Method:

1. Take a Ziploc bag of gallon size. Add a quarter cup of olive oil, chicken, lemon juice, garlic, oregano, red wine vinegar, pepper, and salt and combine them well. Keep them as it is to marinate for at least twenty minutes or up to an hour. Take the bag occasionally and turn it. Once the time is over, take the chicken and drain it from the marinade. You can discard the marinade.
2. Now, take a large-sized skillet and heat two tbsps. of olive oil in it. Keep the flame at medium-high. Add the chicken. Cook it thoroughly and flip it once. You should cook each side for about four minutes. Before you dice the chicken into smaller pieces, let it cool.
3. Make the cucumber salad. For this, combine the cucumber with the rest of the ingredients in a bowl and mix them well. Once done, set the bowl aside.
4. Make the tzatziki sauce. For this, too, combine all the ingredients in a bowl. Drizzle olive oil on top after seasoning with pepper and salt. Mix them all and then put the sauce in the refrigerator for about ten minutes or more. This will allow the flavors to mix. Set it aside.

5. Take a large-sized saucepan and add two cups of water in it. Follow the instructions mentioned on the packet of rice to cook it. Once done, set the rice aside as well.
6. Once the rice has cooled down, scoop it into the meal prep containers equally. Then, top the rice with the cucumber salad, chicken, tzatziki sauce, and tomatoes.

Chapter 7:
Grocery Shopping Tips for Meal Preppers

Yes, I get it that you all have a busy routine, and sparing time for meal prepping and planning might seem tough. But believe me when I say it that if you devote at least ten minutes of your time daily to planning, you will actually save yourself twenty minutes of loss later. To make the task easier, here are some grocery shopping tips from me to you that are going to make meal prepping so much easier than it was before.

Stick to One Supermarket

When you stick to one single supermarket for your grocery shopping, you literally memorize every corner of it, and you know where everything is kept. In this way, you don't have to wander aimlessly searching for the product you are looking for. You should also get to know everyone who works at the supermarket. If you build a good relationship with them, there can be days when you can take the help of that friendship, for example, by asking them to do an emergency delivery for you.

Make a Store Map of Your Own

Take an 8 by 10 paper and draw a grid on it. This will be easier if you take pictures of the items you buy and the racks they are kept on. This will also make budgeting easier. Now, in that grid, make your own aisle numbers for the grocery store. Also, in each aisle, note down the products that you usually purchase from there. Don't forget to leave some extra space for noting down all those products which you buy but not on a regular basis. And here is the most important tip – list the meals that you have planned to prep this week at the top of this list.

Have a Digital Meal List

There will be times when, despite so many recipes, you will feel clueless as to what to cook. That is why you need to adopt a new practice. Make a list of meals you want to cook beforehand and keep that list stored digitally. You can categorize the meals based on their nutrient content and in this way, you will be able to maintain a balanced diet or even adjust the nutrient levels whenever you want. You can also have different folders for appetizers, snacks, side dishes, and main courses. This list can be a work in progress so that whenever you come across a new recipe, you can add it to the list. Also, make it a promise to yourself to add one new recipe every month.

Be Aware of the Sales

Grocery stores sometimes have amazing sales, and you need to be aware of them so that you can take full benefit of such occasions. And here too, planning is the key. You can check for offers online or have a look at the supermarket flyers. If you notice that the sale is on certain selective items, then you can tweak your meal plan accordingly and save a lot of money.

planning, and if you follow the steps that I have mentioned, you should be a meal prep ninja by the end of the month.

Finally, if you found this book useful in any way, a review on Amazon is always appreciated!

Conclusion

Thank you for making it through to the end of *Meal Prep for Beginners: A Complete Meal Prep Cookbook – Your Essential Guide To Losing Weight and Saving Time – Many Quick and Easy Recipes, 30 Day Meal Plan to Weight Loss, And Healthy Meals To Prep and Go!*, let's hope it was informative and able to provide you with all of the tools you need to achieve your goals whatever they may be.

The next step is to start planning. Yes, do it today. Eating healthy does not have to be difficult when you have such amazing options. Meal prepping is a real life savior. Not to mention, you are eating homemade food at all times so adieu all those junk you had been eating earlier. I wrote this book with the aim of making meal prep easier for beginners. There are recipes that hardly take ten minutes, and there are also elaborate recipes that are perfect for a family night.

The aim of the book is to provide a comprehensive approach to meal prepping. So, no more getting late for work in the morning or skipping breakfast because healthy meals are waiting for you in the fridge. But as I have said countless times before, the key to mastering meal prepping is efficient